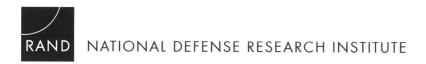 NATIONAL DEFENSE RESEARCH INSTITUTE

T0122976

Quality of Care for PTSD and Depression in the Military Health System

Final Report

Kimberly A. Hepner, Carol P. Roth, Elizabeth M. Sloss,
Susan M. Paddock, Praise O. Iyiewuare, Martha J. Timmer,
Harold Alan Pincus

Prepared for Defense Centers of Excellence for Psychological Health
and Traumatic Brain Injury

For more information on this publication, visit www.rand.org/t/RR1542

Library of Congress Cataloging-in-Publication Data is available for this publication.
ISBN: 978-0-8330-9713-2

Support RAND
Make a tax-deductible charitable contribution at
www.rand.org/giving/contribute

www.rand.org

Preface

The U.S. Department of Defense (DoD) strives to maintain a physically and psychologically healthy, mission-ready force, and the care provided by the Military Health System (MHS) is critical to meeting this goal. Given the rates of posttraumatic stress disorder (PTSD) and depression among U.S. service members, attention has been directed to ensuring the quality and availability of programs and services targeting these and other psychological health (PH) conditions. Understanding the quality of care for PTSD and depression is an important step toward future efforts to improve care across the MHS, including ongoing quality monitoring, quality improvement initiatives, and supporting alternative payment models (e.g., value-based purchasing).

To help determine whether the service members with PTSD or depression are receiving evidence-based care and whether there are disparities in care quality by branch of service, geographic region, and service member characteristics (e.g., gender, age, pay grade, race/ethnicity, deployment history), DoD's Defense Centers of Excellence for Psychological Health and Traumatic Brain Injury (DCoE) asked the RAND Corporation to conduct a review of the administrative data and medical records of service members diagnosed with PTSD and/or depression and to recommend areas on which the MHS could focus its efforts to continuously improve the quality of care provided to all service members. Analyses focus on the quality of care delivered to active-component service members with PTSD or depression, restricted to service members who did not separate from the military or deploy during a one-year observation period. Preliminary analyses of clinical symptom data are also included. This document represents the final report and deliverable for the project. A series of online appendixes are available from the report's web page: www.rand.org/t/RR1542.

This report should be of interest to MHS and Defense Health Agency administrators responsible for ensuring excellence in health care, MHS personnel who provide care for service members with PTSD or depression, and DoD health care beneficiaries. It should also be useful to those responsible for monitoring the quality of that care and developing evidence-based quality measures to improve care for service members and individuals with PTSD or depression in other health systems.

This research was sponsored by DCoE and conducted within the Forces and Resources Policy Center of the RAND National Defense Research Institute, a federally funded research and development center sponsored by the Office of the Secretary of Defense, the Joint Staff, the Unified Combatant Commands, the Navy, the Marine Corps, the defense agencies, and the defense Intelligence Community.

For more information on the RAND Forces and Resources Policy Center, see www.rand.org/nsrd/ndri/centers/frp or contact the director (contact information is provided on the web page).

Contents

Figures

Tables

Summary

This report represents the third in a series of RAND reports about the quality of care for PTSD and depression in the MHS. At the request of DoD, the RAND Corporation initiated a project in 2012 to (1) provide a descriptive baseline assessment of the extent to which providers in the MHS implement care consistent with clinical practice guidelines (CPGs) for PTSD and depression, and (2) examine the relationship between guideline-concordant care and clinical outcomes for these conditions. This report builds on two previous RAND reports, one that presented a set of quality measures developed for care provided to active-component service members with PTSD and depression (Hepner et al., 2015), and another that described characteristics of active-component service members who received care for PTSD or depression from the MHS and assessed the quality of care provided for PTSD and depression using quality measures based on 2012–2013 administrative data (Hepner et al., 2016).

This report provides a more comprehensive assessment of MHS outpatient care for active-component service members with PTSD and depression by including an expanded set of quality measures and using two new sources of data, medical records and symptom questionnaires. As in Phase I, we focus in this report on active-compo-

Table S.1
Quality Measures for Patients with PTSD and Patients with Depression

Measure No.	PTSD	Depression
	Assessment	
A1	Percentage of PTSD patients with a new treatment episode with assessment of symptoms with PCL within 30 days	Percentage of depression patients with a new treatment episode with assessment of symptoms with PHQ-9 within 30 days
A2	Percentage of PTSD patients with a new treatment episode assessed for depression within 30 days	Percentage of depression patients with a new treatment episode assessed for manic/hypomanic behaviors within 30 days
A3	Percentage of PTSD patients with a new treatment episode assessed for suicide risk at same visit	Percentage of depression patients with a new treatment episode assessed for suicide risk at same visit[a]

Table S.1—Continued

Measure No.	PTSD	Depression
	Assessment	
A4	Percentage of PTSD patients with a new treatment episode assessed for recent substance use within 30 days	Percentage of depression patients with a new treatment episode assessed for recent substance use within 30 days
	Treatment	
T1	Percentage of PTSD patients with symptom assessment with PCL during 4-month measurement period	Percentage of depression patients with symptom assessment with PHQ-9 during 4-month measurement period[a]
T3	Percentage of patient contacts of PTSD patients with SI with appropriate follow-up (PTSD-T3)	Percentage of patient contacts of depression patients with SI with appropriate follow-up (Depression-T3)
T5	Percentage of PTSD patients with a newly prescribed SSRI/SNRI with an adequate trial ($\geq$ 60 days)	Percentage of depression patients with a newly prescribed antidepressant with a trial of 12 weeks (T5a) or 6 months (T5b)[a]
T6	Percentage of PTSD patients newly prescribed an SSRI/SNRI with follow-up visit within 30 days	Percentage of depression patients newly prescribed an antidepressant with follow-up visit within 30 days
T7	Percentage of PTSD patients who receive evidence-based psychotherapy for PTSD	Percentage of depression patients who receive evidence-based psychotherapy for depression
T8	Percentage of PTSD patients with a new treatment episode who received any psychotherapy within the first 4 months	Percentage of depression patients with a new treatment episode who received any psychotherapy within the first 4 months
T9	Percentage of PTSD patients with a new treatment episode with 4 psychotherapy visits or 2 evaluation and management visits in the first 8 weeks	Percentage of depression patients with a new treatment episode with 4 psychotherapy visits or 2 evaluation and management visits in the first 8 weeks
T10	Percentage of PTSD patients (PCL score > 43) with response to treatment (5-point reduction in PCL score) at 6 months	Percentage of depression patients (PHQ-9 score > 9) with response to treatment (50% reduction in PHQ-9 score) at 6 months[a]
T12	Percentage of PTSD patients (PCL score > 43) in PTSD-symptom remission (PCL score < 28) at 6 months	Percentage of depression patients (PHQ-9 score > 9) in depression-symptom remission (PHQ-9 score < 5) at 6 months[a]
T14	Percentage of PTSD patients with a new treatment episode with improvement in functional status at 6 months	Percentage of depression patients with a new treatment episode with improvement in functional status at 6 months
T15	Percentage of psychiatric inpatient hospital discharges of patients with PTSD with follow-up in 7 days (T15a) or 30 days (T15b)[a]	Percentage of psychiatric inpatient hospital discharges of patients with depression with follow-up in 7 days (T15a) or 30 days (T15b)[a]

NOTE: PCL = PTSD Checklist; PHQ-9 = Patient Health Questionnaire, 9-item; SSRI = selective serotonin reuptake inhibitor; SNRI = serotonin and norepinephrine reuptake inhibitor.

[a] NQF-endorsed measure.

nent service members to increase the likelihood that the care they received was pro-vided or paid for by the MHS, rather than other sources of health care. Data from all three data sources were analyzed for the 2013–2014 time period—more recent than the time period used for the analyses in our previous report, which was 2012–2013 (Hepner et al., 2016). We describe the characteristics of active-component service members who received care for PTSD or depression from the MHS in 2013–2014 based on administrative data. We also assess the quality of care provided for PTSD and depression using quality measures based on three data sources for 2013–2014. Finally, we explore the use of symptom scores in the MHS and the relationship between adher-ence to guideline-concordant care and symptom scores; these analyses were limited to Army personnel who were seen in military treatment facility (MTF) behavioral health clinics, due to data availability.

Selecting Quality Measures for PTSD and Depression Care

Quality measures provide a way to measure how well health care is being delivered. Quality measures are applied by operationalizing aspects of care recommended by CPGs using administrative data, medical records, clinical registries, patient or clinician surveys, and other data sources. Such measures provide information about the health care system and highlight areas in which providers can take action to make health care safer and more equitable (National Quality Forum [NQF], 2017a and 2017b). Qual-ity measures usually incorporate operationally defined numerators and denominators, and scores are typically presented as the percentage of eligible patients who received the

Figure S.1
Timing of Cohort Entry and Computation of 12-Month Observation Period

Cohort selection window

January 2013   June 2013   June 2014

Range of dates for observation period

Two examples:

12-month observation period (February 12, 2013–February 12, 2014)
Patient A:
PTSD
Diagnosis on
February 12, 2013

12-month observation period (April 26, 2013–April 26, 2014)
Patient B:
Depression
Diagnosis on
April 26, 2013

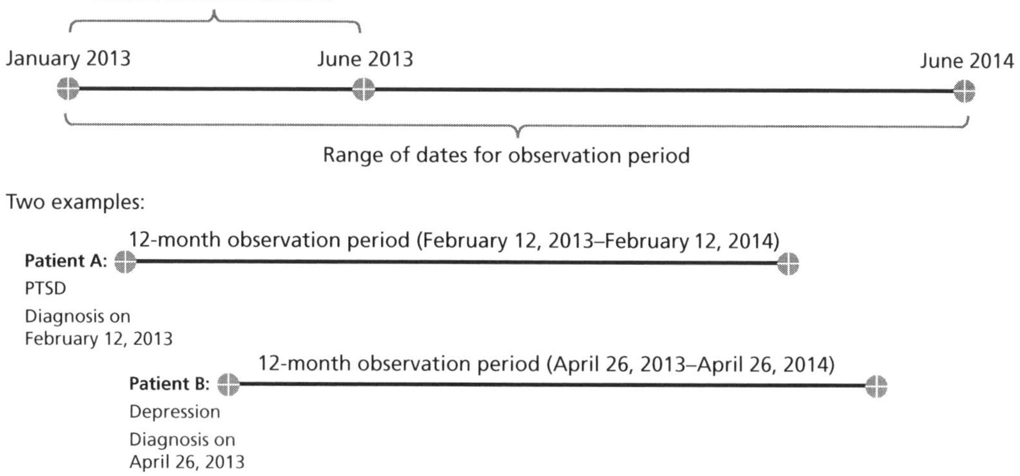

RAND RR1542-S.1

recommended care (e.g., percentage of patients who receive timely outpatient follow-up after inpatient discharge). Based on previous work conducted by RAND, we selected 15 quality measures for PTSD and 15 quality measures for depression as the focus of this report. These measures are described briefly in Table S.1, with detailed technical specifications provided in Appendixes A and B.[1] These measures assess care described in the U.S. Department of Veterans Affairs (VA)/DoD CPG for the Management of Major Depressive Disorder (MDD) (VA and DoD, 2009) and Management of Post-Traumatic Stress Disorder and Acute Stress Reaction (VA and DoD, 2010), including assessment of patients starting a new treatment episode, follow-up of positive suicidal ideation, adequate medication management, receipt of psychotherapy, receipt of a minimal number of visits associated with a first-line treatment (either psychotherapy or medication management), monitoring of symptoms over time, response to treatment, and follow-up after hospital discharge for a mental health condition. During this study, these two VA/DoD guidelines were in the process of being updated. The updated VA/DoD MDD guideline (VA and DoD, 2016) was made available shortly before this report was released, but the updated PTSD guideline had not yet been published.

Methods and Data Sources

We used three types of data for our analyses: administrative, medical record, and symptom questionnaire.

Administrative Data

We used administrative data that contained records on all inpatient and outpatient health care encounters for MHS beneficiaries in an MTF (i.e., direct care) or by civilian providers paid for by TRICARE (i.e., purchased care). To describe and evaluate care for PTSD and depression, we identified a cohort of patients who received care for PTSD and a cohort who received care for depression. Service members were eligible for the PTSD or depression cohort if they had at least one outpatient visit or inpatient stay with a primary or secondary diagnosis for PTSD or depression, respectively, during the first six months of 2013 (January 1–June 30, 2013) in either direct care or purchased care (Figure S.1). The 12-month observation period starts with the date of the qualifying visit (first visit for PTSD or depression in the cohort selection window) and occurs between January 1, 2013, and June 30, 2014, but the exact start and end dates differ by patient.

The criteria for selecting these diagnostic cohorts were the following:

---

[1] Available online with this report: http://www.rand.org/pubs/research_reports/RR1542.html.

- *Active-Component Service Members*—The patient must have been an active-component service member during the entire 12-month observation period.
- *Received Care for PTSD or Depression*—Service members could enter the PTSD or depression cohort if they had at least one outpatient visit or inpatient stay (direct or purchased care) with a PTSD or depression diagnosis (primary or secondary) during January through June 2013. We did not limit the depression cohort to MDD, but rather included other depression diagnoses as well to include codes used to identify depression for denominators for NQF-endorsed measures.[2] Also, while the recently updated VA/DoD MDD guideline notes that it does not address non-MDD depression, it recommends that its principles be strongly considered when treating other depressive disorders (VA and DoD, 2016).
- *Engaged with and Eligible for MHS Care*—Service members were eligible for a cohort if they had received a minimum of one inpatient stay or two outpatient visits for any diagnosis (i.e., related or not related to PTSD or depression) within the MHS (either direct or purchased care) during the 12-month observation period following the index visit. In addition, service members must have been eligible for TRICARE benefits during the entire 12-month observation period. Members who deployed or separated from the service during the 12-month period were excluded.

Using these criteria, we identified 14,654 service members for the PTSD cohort and 30,496 for the depression cohort. A total of 6,322 service members were in both cohorts, representing 43.1 percent of the PTSD cohort and 20.7 percent of the depression cohort. Therefore, the two cohorts together represent a total of 38,828 unique service members.

To describe the quality of care for PTSD and depression delivered by the MHS, we computed scores for each quality measure. For measures based on administrative data, we also examined variations in quality measure scores by service branch (Army, Air Force, Marine Corps, Navy) and TRICARE region (North, South, West, Overseas). In addition, we examined variations across service member characteristics, including age, race/ethnicity, gender, pay grade, and history of deployment at time of cohort entry.

Administrative data are particularly well suited for assessing care provision and quality across a large population, although such data do have limitations. For example, they do not include clinical detail documented in chart notes, including whether a patient refused a particular treatment or whether an evidence-based psychotherapy was delivered.

---

[2]   ICD-9 codes for depression: 296.20–296.26, 296.30–296.36, 293.83, 296.90, 296.99, 298.0, 300.4, 309.1, and 311.

Medical Record Data

Medical record review (MRR) was conducted on a stratified, random sample of service members from the PTSD and depression cohorts, limiting the sample to service members who received only direct care during the observation period. This limitation was based on the fact that medical records documenting purchased care were not accessible for abstraction. The source of medical record data was AHLTA, the electronic health record used by the MTFs to document outpatient care. Medical record review incorporated a hybrid methodology where administrative data were used to identify service members within the MRR sample with characteristics relevant to quality measure eligibility.

To select the MRR sample, the study population was restricted to the 16,173 service members in the Army, Air Force, Marine Corps, and Navy[3,4] who received only direct care during their observation year. For purposes of yielding two distinct MRR samples for PTSD and depression, we randomly assigned each of the 1,616 service members with both PTSD and depression diagnoses to either the PTSD or depression cohort.[5] From each of these groups, we drew a random sample of 400 service members. Service members with a new treatment episode (NTE) on the first day of cohort entry were oversampled to ensure the sample contained a sufficient number of service members eligible for the MRR measures focusing on NTEs.[6] The sample was also stratified to ensure that service members were represented by branch, region, and by having both PTSD and depression versus having one of these conditions. Sampling weights for estimating the measure scores of the NTE and all-cohort quality measures were applied to account for the stratified sampling plan. For details of the MRR methods, see Appendix C.[7]

Medical record data provide a level of clinical detail not available from other data sources. However, the comprehensiveness of medical record data depends on the providers' documenting all care that was provided. Data collection from the medical record is also time-intensive and expensive compared to collection of other types of data. In this project, time and budget constraints led to a reduction in the planned

---

[3]   Coast Guard service members were not sampled since their relatively small proportion in the service member population would not allow for a sufficient number of them to be sampled to yield Coast Guard–specific estimates.

[4]   Those with missing region are excluded from the sampled population.

[5]   The probability of random assignment to the PTSD cohort is higher (0.70 versus 0.30), since the proportion of the cohort with both PTSD and depression at the time of cohort entry is higher for the PTSD (32 percent) than for the depression cohort (12 percent).

[6]   NTEs were limited to those that occurred on Day 1 of cohort entry (representing 96 and 97 percent of the total NTEs for PTSD and depression, respectively) to maximize the length of the observation period. Those with NTEs occurring only after Day 1 of cohort entry (e.g., a patient could have entered the cohort in ongoing treatment and then had a three-month clean period with no treatment, followed by receiving treatment again) were not sampled.

[7]   Available online with this report: http://www.rand.org/pubs/research_reports/RR1542.html.

medical record data collection and, therefore, a reduction in the number of quality measures that could be computed from this data source. The "dropped" measures were computed using symptom questionnaire data instead (as described next).

Symptom Questionnaire Data

Data from symptom questionnaires are available from a dedicated data collection system within MHS. The system, known as the Behavioral Health Data Portal (BHDP), has been in operation since September 2013 in all of Army's behavioral health clinics, and implementation in other service branches is under way. The BHDP is an easy-to-use and secure web-based system for collecting behavioral health symptom data directly from patients (Hoge et al., 2015) but is separate from the electronic health record where the scores must be entered manually. Our analyses focused on PTSD and depression symptom questionnaires—the PTSD Checklist (PCL) for PTSD, and the Patient Health Questionnaire-9 (PHQ-9) for depression. Each PCL or PHQ-9 score and the date completed were linked to the administrative data records of individuals in the PTSD and depression cohorts. These symptom scores were used to compute scores for selected quality measures and for descriptive and multivariate analyses. These analyses were restricted to subgroups with access to the BHDP (e.g., Army, direct care only, behavioral health encounters). When considered together, these factors mean that the symptom questionnaire data represent only a subset of the service members with PTSD or depression, which may not be representative of all service members with PTSD or depression.

The symptom questionnaire data collected through the BHDP offer a way to track clinical outcomes of treatment for PH conditions delivered by providers at MTFs. Symptom data are captured in structured fields, making the data easily accessible. Despite these advantages, the data have limitations: BHDP is not directly linked to AHLTA, and the provider must therefore either enter the proper diagnosis for the system to know which symptom questionnaire should be administered and how often or change how often the questionnaire should be administered directly; at the time of this study, symptom questionnaires were completed within the BHDP only by patients seen in behavioral health specialty care at an MTF (i.e., direct care). In addition, an unbiased comparison of outcome measures, including symptom scores, across groups should be adjusted for differences in severity, so one group does not appear to have worse outcomes simply because that group's patients have greater pre-existing severity. Furthermore, symptom scores of subgroups of service members (e.g., those with initial and six-month follow-up scores within the observation period) may not be representative of all service members with PTSD or depression, or of all with a symptom score. Note that the symptom questionnaire data were used in two separate analyses, as the basis for computing quality measure scores and in regression analyses.

Characteristics of Service Members Diagnosed with PTSD and Depression, Their Care Settings, and Services Received

Demographic Characteristics

The majority of service members in the PTSD cohort were white, non-Hispanic, male, with nearly half the cohort between 25 and 34 years of age (see Table 3.1 in Chapter Three). About a third of the PTSD cohort resided in TRICARE South, with another third located in TRICARE West and one-fifth in TRICARE North. The depression cohort exhibited similar characteristics, except a higher percentage of the depression cohort was female, younger, and never married.

Army soldiers represented 69 and 56 percent of the PTSD and depression cohorts, respectively (see Table 3.2 in Chapter Three). Enlisted service members represented nearly 90 percent of both cohorts. Approximately 50 percent (PTSD) and 60 percent (depression) of service members in the cohorts had ten or fewer years of service. In the PTSD cohort, almost 90 percent of service members had at least one deployment at the time of cohort entry, while in the depression cohort, 68 percent had been deployed.

Care Settings and Diagnoses

Patients in the PTSD and depression cohorts received much of their care at MTFs (over 90 percent had at least some direct care); yet 30 percent of patients in the PTSD cohort and 22 percent in the depression cohort received at least some purchased care. Nearly 60 percent of all primary diagnoses coded for encounters (and presumed to be the primary reason for the encounter) in both direct care and purchased care were for non-PH diagnoses. The most common co-occurring PH conditions in both cohorts were adjustment and anxiety disorders, as well as sleep disorders or symptoms. More than half of the PTSD cohort had co-occurring depression at any point during the 12-month observation period.[8]

Approximately two-thirds of patients in the depression cohort and three-fourths of patients in the PTSD cohort received care associated with a cohort diagnosis (coded in any position, primary or secondary) from MTF mental health specialty settings, while almost half of each cohort had cohort-related diagnoses documented at MTF primary care clinics. Further, patients saw many provider types for care associated with a cohort diagnosis (primary or secondary). About half of patients in both the PTSD and depression cohorts saw primary care providers, and high percentages saw psychiatrists (47 percent for PTSD; 40 percent for depression), clinical psychologists (46 percent for PTSD; 33 percent for depression), and social workers (47 percent for PTSD; 34 percent for depression) for this care. The median number of unique providers seen by cohort patients during the observation year at encounters with a cohort diagnosis

---

[8]   Co-occurring diagnoses examined over the entire 12-month observation period; overlap between the two cohorts was based on diagnoses at cohort entry, limited to the first six months of 2013. Therefore, the prevalence of comorbid PTSD/depression may be higher than the overlap between the two cohorts.

(coded in any position) was three for PTSD and two for depression. When considering all outpatient encounters (for any reason), the median number of unique providers was 14 for those in the PTSD cohort and 12 for those in the depression cohort. This suggests that patients with PTSD or depression may be seen by multiple providers across primary and specialty care, highlighting the importance of understanding these patterns to inform efforts to improve coordination of care for these patients.

Assessment and Treatment Characteristics

Approximately 20 percent of each cohort had an inpatient hospitalization for any reason (i.e., medical or psychiatric), but a substantial proportion of these inpatient

Figure S.2
PTSD Quality Measure Scores, 2013–2014

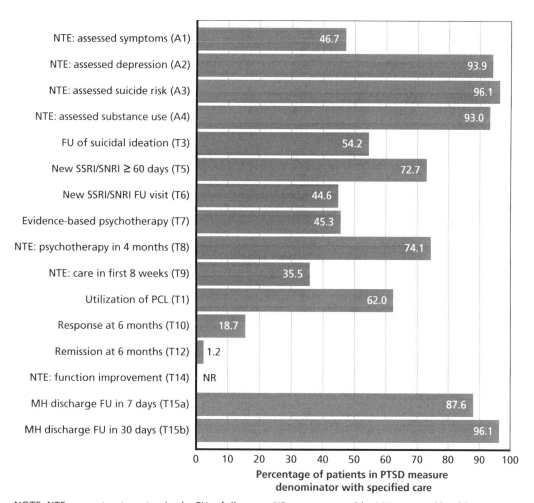

NOTE: NTE = new treatment episode; FU = follow-up; NR = not reportable; MH = mental health.
RAND RR1542-S.2

Figure S.3
Depression Quality Measure Scores, 2013–2014

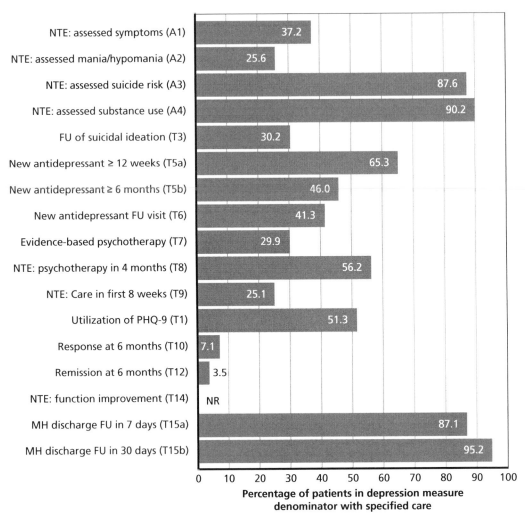

RAND RR1542-S.3

stays had the cohort condition listed as a primary or secondary diagnosis (66 percent for PTSD; 60 percent for depression). For inpatient hospitalizations that had a primary diagnosis of PTSD or depression, the median length of stay per admission was 25 days for patients in the PTSD cohort and seven days for patients in the depression cohort. Utilization of outpatient care for any reason was high, with medians of 40 and 31 visits for PTSD and depression during the one-year observation period, respectively, a finding possibly related to the large number of unique providers seen. Most of these visits were for conditions unrelated to the cohort diagnosis, with only ten and four of these visits having PTSD and depression as the primary diagnosis, respectively.

Over three-quarters of patients in the PTSD cohort and more than two-thirds of the depression cohort received psychiatric diagnostic evaluation or psychological testing, while other testing and assessment methods, including neuropsychological testing and health and behavior assessment, were used with much lower frequency. A high percentage of patients received at least one psychotherapy visit (individual, group, or family therapy)—approximately 91 percent of the PTSD cohort and 83 percent of the depression cohort. For both cohorts, individual therapy was received by a much higher percentage of patients than group therapy, while family therapy was received by a much smaller percentage. If receiving psychotherapy, patients in the PTSD cohort received an average of 19 psychotherapy sessions (across therapy modalities), while approximately 15 of these visits had a PTSD diagnosis (in any position). Patients in the depression cohort received an average of 14 psychotherapy sessions, of which approximately nine visits had a depression diagnosis (in any position).

More than 85 percent of service members in both cohorts filled at least one prescription for psychotropic medication during the observation year. Antidepressants were filled by the highest percentage of both cohorts (77 and 79 percent of the PTSD and depression cohorts, respectively), while stimulants were filled by the smallest percentage (11 percent in both cohorts). Of note is the finding that about 33 percent of the PTSD cohort and 25 percent of the depression cohort filled at least one benzodiazepine prescription. In addition, 57 and 50 percent of the PTSD and depression cohorts, respectively, filled at least one opioid prescription. Patients in the PTSD and depression cohorts also filled prescriptions for multiple psychotropic medications from different classes or within the same medication class. About 25 and 29 percent of the PTSD and depression cohorts, respectively, had prescriptions from two different classes, while 42 percent of the PTSD cohort and 26 percent of the depression cohort filled prescriptions from three or more classes of medication. These results indicate that many patients in both cohorts received prescriptions for multiple psychotropic medications.

Quality of Care for PTSD and Depression

Figures S.2 and S.3 summarize our overall findings for each quality measure for the PTSD and depression cohorts, respectively. Each quality measure focuses on the subset of patients who met the eligibility requirements as specified in the measure denominator. Measure scores above 75 percent were considered to be high, and those below 50 percent were considered to be low, although published scores for the same or similar measures in comparable populations also informed our assessment. Starting with care for PTSD, approximately 47 percent of active-component service members in the MRR sample with a new treatment episode (NTE) of PTSD had an assessment of symptom severity with the PCL, but 93 to 96 percent had an assessment of depression, suicide risk, or recent substance use (Figure S.2). However, 54 percent of PTSD patients in the MRR sample had appropriate follow-up for suicidal ideation. Approximately 73 percent of the PTSD cohort with a new prescription for an SSRI or SNRI filled prescriptions for at least a 60-day supply. Of those who received a new SSRI/SNRI prescription, about 45 percent had a follow-up evaluation and management (E&M) visit within 30 days. Nearly three-quarters of service members in the PTSD cohort with a new treatment episode received some type of psychotherapy within four months. However, less than half (45 percent) of PTSD patients in the MRR sample who had psychotherapy had at least two documented components of evidence-based therapy (EBT). A low proportion (36 percent) received a minimally appropriate level of care for patients entering a new treatment episode, defined as receiving four psychotherapy visits or two E&M visits within the initial eight weeks. Minimal utilization of the PCL for PTSD symptom assessment based on symptom questionnaire data increased from 44 percent in the first four-month interval to 62 percent in the last four-month interval of the observation year. While this increase in rate is encouraging, it is based on symptom questionnaire data limited to the Army and patients seen in behavioral health settings in direct care. Percentages with response to treatment and remission for PTSD in six months were low, at 19 percent and 1 percent, respectively. Again, these percentages with response and remission are to be taken in the context of the data limitations noted above. Improvement in function within six months of a new PTSD or depression diagnosis could not be assessed due to the lack of use in the studied population of standardized tools to evaluate this outcome. Percentages with follow-up after hospitalization for a mental health condition were high: 88 percent within seven days of discharge, and 96 percent within 30 days. For the six PTSD measures based on administrative data scored in 2012–2013, scores in 2013–2014 increased slightly (increase of 1 to 3 percentage points) for five of them.

In the depression cohort, 37 percent in the MRR sample beginning a new treatment episode had a baseline assessment of symptom severity with the PHQ-9 (based on the medical record), and 26 percent had an assessment for behaviors of mania or hypomania, but 88 percent and 90 percent had an assessment for suicide risk and recent substance use, respectively, Figure S.3). A low proportion (30 percent) of patients with depression and suicidal ideation in the MRR sample had appropriate follow-up. Almost two-thirds of service members with a new prescription for an antidepressant medication in the depression cohort filled at least a 12-week supply, and 46 percent filled at least a six-month supply. Among those who filled a new prescription for an antidepressant, 41 percent had a follow-up E&M visit within 30 days. Over half of service members in the depression cohort (56 percent) received psychotherapy within four months of a new treatment episode of depression. However, a low proportion (30 percent) of patients with depression in the MRR sample who had psychotherapy had at least two documented components of cognitive behavioral therapy (CBT). A similar low percentage of 25 percent of service members in the depression cohort received a minimum of four psychotherapy visits or two E&M visits within the first eight weeks of their new depression diagnosis. Rates of utilization of the PHQ-9 to assess depression symptoms increased during each measured increment of the 12-month observation period; by the third (and final) four-month period, minimal PHQ-9 utilization had increased from 36 percent in the first four-month interval to 51 percent during the last four-month interval of the observation year. Percentages with response to treatment and remission for depression in six months were low at 7 percent and 4 percent, respectively. These percentages for depression, as with PTSD, were based on symptom questionnaire data limited to the Army and patients seen in behavioral health settings in direct care. Percentages with follow-up after discharge from a hospitalization for a mental health condition for those with depression were high: 87 percent within seven days of discharge, and 95 percent within 30 days. Six of seven depression measures computed using administrative data had scores in 2013–2014 that increased from those in 2012–2013, but these increases were small (i.e., increases ranged from 1 to 4 percentage points).

While it is often difficult, or not appropriate, to directly compare results from other health care systems or studies or related measures, prior published results for these measures (or highly related measures) are presented in this report to provide important context to guide interpretation. These comparisons serve to highlight areas where the MHS may outperform other health care systems (e.g., in timely follow-up after inpatient mental health discharge), perform at a comparable level (e.g., adequate trial of antidepressant therapy for patients with depression with a new prescription) or that may be high priorities for improvement (e.g., receipt of adequate care in the first eight weeks of a new treatment episode). It should be noted that although the MHS should work toward improvement on all of these measures, the results presented provide a preliminary guide for prioritizing targets for routine measurement and improvement. The MHS could select high-priority targets based on those measures with lower scores (e.g., receipt of adequate care in the first eight weeks of a new treatment episode) or measures that assess processes that could be particularly high-risk for service members if not completed (e.g., follow-up after suicide risk).

Variations in Administrative Data Measure Scores

Using 2013–2014 administrative data, we conducted an assessment of the variation in measure scores by service branch, TRICARE region, and service member characteristics, including age, gender, race/ethnicity, pay grade, and deployment history as we had conducted on 2012–2013 administrative data. Most of the variations in measure scores persisted between the two years (see Tables 4.18 and 4.19 in Chapter Four and Tables 5.18 and 5.19 in Chapter Five for PTSD and depression results, respectively). The largest differences occurred by branch of service, TRICARE region, pay grade, and age. For branch of service, follow-up within seven days after a mental health hospitalization

(T15a) varied by up to 16 percent and 15 percent in the PTSD and depression cohorts, respectively. For TRICARE region, follow-up within 30 days after a new prescription of SSRI/ SNRI (PTSD-T6) varied up to 12 percent in the PTSD cohort. For pay grade, percentages with adequate filled prescriptions for SSRI/SNRI for PTSD (PTSD-T5) and antidepressants for depression (Depression-T5a and -T5b) varied by up to 8, 24, and 30 percent, respectively. For age, percentages with adequate filled prescriptions for SSRI/SNRI for PTSD (PTSD-T5) and antidepressants for depression (Depression-T5a and -T5b) varied by up to 10, 18, and 24 percent, respectively. The depression measure scores suggest even more variation across subgroups than the PTSD measures. In targeting areas for quality improvement activities, differences in measure scores based on service branch, TRICARE region, pay grade, and age should be considered. For example, quality measures with particularly large variations in scores or variations across multiple characteristics could be the first measures selected for ongoing monitoring and quality improvement.

Use of Symptom Questionnaires in MTFs

Since 2012, Army behavioral health clinics have collected self-reported outcome data using standardized symptom questionnaires using the BHDP. Army intends to use these symptom scores to inform both clinical care and assessment of patient outcomes. Of the 8,510 Army personnel in our PTSD cohort who had two or more mental health specialty care visits, 45 percent completed two or more PCLs over their 12-month observation period in 2013–2014. Of the 13,746 Army personnel in the depression cohort who had two or more mental health specialty care visits, one-third completed two or more PHQ-9s in their 12-month observation period in 2013–2014.

We assessed the use of the BHDP for completing the PCL and PHQ-9 on a monthly basis from February 2013 through June 2014. We found the overall PCL completion rate in the PTSD cohort and overall PHQ-9 completion rate in the depression cohort increased steadily in 2013–2014 to 21.5 and 17.2 per 100 MH specialty visits, respectively, in June 2014. Although these rates are relatively low, they represent a time period early in the use of the BHDP system when providers and patients were new to the system, and completion rates would be expected to continue to increase over time. Notably, the completion rate was consistently higher for the PCL by the PTSD cohort than for the PHQ-9 for the depression cohort throughout the entire period.

Symptom Scores: Change over Time and Link to Process Measures

In examining changes in symptom scores over time, we found in the PTSD and depression cohorts that symptom scores improved from the initial score to six months later among Army soldiers with two or more mental health specialty visits by a statistically significant, but not a clinically meaningful, amount. Reductions in symptom scores were larger for the subset of Army soldiers in a new treatment episode and/or with initial PCL scores greater than or equal to 50 points or initial PHQ-9 scores greater than or equal to 10 points. We did not detect significant associations between receiving recommended care, as specified in the PTSD and depression quality measures, and improvements in patient symptoms at six months after the initial score. A limitation of these analyses is that the data reflect the subset with continued engagement and reassessment in behavioral health specialty care. For example, patients with multiple behavioral health specialty care visits may improve and complete treatment in less than five months. This subgroup would not be reflected in these results because its members would not be in treatment to be assessed at the six-month point in time. However, similar results were found for examining symptom score change from the initial score to three months later. Though we weight our analysis to account for differences between those with versus without reassessments, the weights adjust only for observed characteristics at the time of the initial score. Finally, while these analyses are preliminary, they demonstrate the potential value of routinely collected data on patient outcomes. More research on particular subgroups may demonstrate clinically meaningful improvement within six months (e.g., service members with more severe symptoms at the time of the initial score).

Policy Implications

PTSD and depression are frequent diagnoses in active-duty service members (Blakeley and Jansen, 2013). If not appropriately identified and treated, these conditions may cause morbidity that would represent a potentially significant threat to the readiness of the force. Assessments of the current quality of care for PTSD and depression in the MHS are an important step toward future efforts to improve care. Based on our findings, we offer several recommendations related to measuring, monitoring, and improving the quality of care received by patients with PTSD or depression in the MHS. These are high-level recommendations that would be implemented most efficiently in an enterprise-wide manner.

Recommendation 1. Improve the Quality of Care Delivered by the Military Health System for Psychological Health Conditions by Immediately Focusing on Specific Care Processes Identified for Improvement

The results presented in this report, combined with the results presented in the Phase I report (Hepner et al., 2016), represent perhaps the largest assessments of quality of outpatient care for PTSD and depression for service members ever conducted. We concluded that while there are some strengths, quality of care for psychological health conditions delivered by the MHS should be improved. For both PTSD and depression, we observed low percentages (36 percent and 25 percent, respectively) of adequate initial care in the first eight weeks following an initial diagnosis (either four psychotherapy or two medication management visits) and of receiving a medication management visit within 30 days of starting a new medication (45 percent and 41 percent, respectively). This suggests that the MHS should identify procedures that would ensure service members receive an adequate intensity of treatment and follow-up when beginning treatment. Further, we found the MHS had high percentages for screening for suicide risk. However, providing adequate follow-up for those with suicide risk could be improved given that a low proportion (30 percent) of service members with depression who were identified as having suicide risk in a new treatment episode received adequate follow-up (i.e., assessment for plan and access to lethal means, referral or follow-up appointment, and discussion of limitation of access to lethal means if access assessment was positive or was not done). Appropriate follow-up care for suicide risk is an essential component of reducing the rate of suicide among service members. Finally, given the extensive and complex patterns of psychopharmacologic prescribing, further analysis of these patterns and development and implementation of quality monitoring and improvement strategies should be a high priority.

Recommendation 2. Expand Efforts to Routinely Assess Quality of Psychological Health Care

Recommendation 2a. Establish an Enterprise-Wide Performance Measurement, Monitoring, and Improvement System That Includes High-Priority Standardized Measures to Assess Care for Psychological Health Conditions

Currently, there is no coordinated enterprise-wide (direct and purchased care) system for monitoring the quality of PH care. A separate system for PH is not required; high-priority PH measures could be integrated into an enterprise-wide system that assesses care across medical and psychiatric conditions. The review of the MHS (DoD, 2014c) highlighted the need for such a system as well. Although the quality measures presented in this report highlight areas for improvement, quality measures for other PH conditions should be considered for reporting (e.g., care for alcohol use disorders). Furthermore, an infrastructure is necessary to support the implementation of quality measures for PH conditions on a local and enterprise-wide basis, and to support other activities, including monitoring performance, conducting analysis of measure scores, validating the process-outcome link for each measure, and evaluating the effect of quality improvement strategies. This function could be executed by a DoD center focused on psychological health (e.g., DCoE) or additional psychological health quality measures could be integrated into ongoing efforts conducted by DoD Health Affairs.

Recommendation 2b. Routinely Report Quality Measure Scores for PH Conditions Internally, Enterprise-Wide, and Publicly to Support and Incentivize Ongoing Quality Improvement and Facilitate Transparency

Routine internal reporting of quality measure results (MHS-wide and at the service and MTF level) provides valuable information to identify gaps in quality, target quality improvement efforts, and evaluate the results of those efforts. The MHS is implementing quality improvement strategies using an "enterprise management approach" and "defining value from the perspective of the patient," including use of systems-approach interventions such as case managers to coordinate care (Woodson, 2016). Analyses of variations in care across service branches, TRICARE regions, or patient characteristics can also guide quality improvement efforts. While Veterans Health Administration (VHA) and civilian health care settings have used monetary incentives for administrators and providers to improve performance, the MHS could provide special recognition in place of financial incentives or provide additional discretionary budget to MTFs for improved performance or maintaining high performance. In addition, reporting of selected quality measures for PH conditions could be required under contracts with purchased care providers (Institute of Medicine, 2010). Quality measures are an essential component of alternative payment models, such as value-based purchasing.

Reporting quality measure results externally provides transparency, which encourages accountability for high-quality care. External reporting could be focused on a more limited set of quality measures that are most tightly linked with outcomes or reported by other health care systems, while a broader set of measures that are descriptive or exploratory could be reported internally. In addition, external reporting allows comparisons with other health care systems that report publicly (though appropriate risk-adjustment is required for outcome measures). Finally, external reporting allows the MHS to demonstrate improvements in performance over time to multiple stakeholders, including service members and other MHS beneficiaries, providers, and policymakers.

In 2016, the MHS and the Defense Health Agency (DHA) launched a public, online quality reporting system (http://www.health.mil/Military-Health-Topics/Access-Cost-Quality-and-Safety) with measure scores by MTF for measures of patient safety, health care outcomes, quality of care, and patient satisfaction and access to care (Military Health System and Defense Health Agency, 2016). The set of HEDIS outpatient measures displayed on the site includes one PH measure: follow-up within seven days and 30 days after mental health discharge. The set of ORYX inpatient measures displayed on the site includes two PH measures: substance use and tobacco treatment.[9] This system could be expanded to include other PH measures and coordinated

---

[9] The ORYX quality measures (also known as the National Hospital Quality Measures) were developed by the Joint Commission for care in the inpatient setting (Joint Commission, 2017). ORYX is not an acronym.

enterprise-wide for monitoring the quality of all direct and purchased care. These are promising efforts that the MHS should continue to expand.

Recommendation 3. Expand Efforts to Monitor and Use Treatment Outcomes for Service Members with Psychological Health Conditions

Recommendation 3a. Integrate Routine Outcome Monitoring for Service Members with PH Conditions as Structured Data in the Medical Record as Part of a Measurement-Based Care Strategy

Routine symptom monitoring for PTSD, depression, and anxiety disorders is now mandated by policy across the MHS (DoD, 2013) using the BHDP (DoD, 2016; DoD and VA, 2014; Department of the Army Headquarters, undated), and the service branches are working toward full implementation of this policy. While encouraging routine symptom monitoring is a positive step, the chief limitation of the BHDP is that it is not electronically linked to the medical record. Because of this, the symptom scores from the BHDP must be entered manually into the medical record by the clinician. As the new medical record system for the MHS is being developed, it would be advantageous to integrate outcome tracking within the medical record. While there are structured, data-mineable fields for symptom questionnaire data currently in AHLTA, this approach does not easily support tracking of patient progress over time—a capability currently included in the BHDP. Further, the MHS should explore how to obtain similar data for patients seen in purchased care.

Recommendation 3b. Monitor Implementation of BHDP Across Services and Evaluate How Providers Use Symptom Data to Inform Clinical Care

We demonstrated the increasing use of the PCL and the PHQ-9 over time during 2013–2014 among Army soldiers with PTSD or depression seen in MTF behavioral health clinics, but also highlighted that the Army can continue to increase the rates of routinely using these measures with patients. Other service branches are now migrating to BHDP. Assessing use of BHDP across all service branches will be important to ensure full implementation occurs. Further, it is important to understand how providers are making decisions in using the BHDP and ensure providers are able to integrate symptom questionnaire information into treatment planning and adjustment, rather than simply entering data because the MHS requires it.

Recommendation 3c. Build Strategies to Effectively Use Outcome Data and Address the Limitations of These Data

The Army's use of BHDP likely represents one of the largest efforts to capture outcomes for patients with PH conditions in the United States, an effort that we highly commend. Results from the outcome quality measures provide a baseline assessment for Army MTF behavioral health clinics and suggest that efforts to monitor and improve treatment outcomes are needed. Our analyses highlighted some of the challenges of using clinic-based assessments of outcomes. A chief limitation of the BHDP is that outcome data are not collected if patients do not return to MTF specialty behavioral health care. Of those with an initial PCL score, 32.6 percent (1,762/5,405) had a PCL score five to seven months later. Of those with an initial PHQ-9 score, 27.6 percent (2,009/7,273) had a PHQ-9 score five to seven months later. Telephone follow-up of patients who did not return to treatment at six months would provide important data about their clinical status at that point in time. Alternatively, this could be integrated into ongoing efforts to assess patient experiences in receiving care, including patient satisfaction, timeliness of care, and interpersonal quality (e.g., felt respected). Further, the BHDP typically captures patients seen in specialty behavioral health care at an MTF and does not include patients who receive their care in primary care clinics (which frequently occurs, particularly for depression) or those who use purchased care for some or all of their care. While AHLTA includes structured, data-mineable fields to capture symptom questionnaire data, AHLTA does not easily support monitoring patient progress over time. Finding ways to collect outcome data routinely across all patients receiving care for psychological health conditions would bolster the representativeness of the data and offer a more complete picture of quality.

Recommendation 4. Investigate the Reasons for Significant Variation in Quality of Care for PH Conditions by Service Branch, Region, and Service Member Characteristics

The 2013–2014 quality measure scores in the current report varied by member and service characteristics in the same ways as our previous 2012–2013 results (Hepner et al., 2016). We found several statistically significant differences in measure scores by service branch, TRICARE region, and service member characteristics, many of which may represent clinically meaningful differences. Understanding and minimizing variations in care by personal characteristic (e.g., gender, race/ethnicity, and geographic region) is important to ensure that care is equitable, one of the six aims of quality of care improvement in the seminal report Crossing the Quality Chasm (Institute of Medicine, 2001). Exploring the structure and processes used by MTFs and staff in high- and low-performing service branches and TRICARE regions may help to identify promising improvement strategies for, and problematic barriers to, providing high-quality care and moving toward the goal of being a high-reliability organization (Woodson, 2016). However, the first step to understanding how to minimize variations and improve quality is to ensure systems are in place to routinely obtain results on high-priority measures.

Summary

This report expands previous RAND research assessing the quality of care provided to active-component service members with PTSD or depression in the MHS. In this report, we analyzed three types of data (administrative, medical record, and symptom questionnaire) to assess performance using 30 quality measures (33 measures, when accounting for scores reported separately within a measure). We also used administrative data to describe patterns of care received by service members with PTSD or depression and examine variations in quality measure scores. Finally, we analyzed symptom questionnaire data to evaluate the relationship between quality of care and patient outcomes. MHS-wide performance across the quality measures was mixed. The MHS demonstrated excellent care in some areas; six measure scores (four for PTSD; two for depression) were at or above 90 percent (assessing PTSD symptom severity and PTSD and depression comorbidity and follow-up after MH hospitalization). In contrast, six PTSD measure scores and nine depression measure scores indicated that fewer than 50 percent of service members received the recommended care. In general, MHS-wide measure scores for PTSD were higher than those for depression. Analyzing variations in administrative data quality measure scores revealed several significant differences, with the largest variations in performance by service branch, TRICARE region, pay grade, and age. These variations are important because they suggest that care is not consistently of high quality for all service members. No significant associations were found between receiving recommended care and improvements in patient symptom scores at six months, but the analyses were limited to a subgroup of patients with continued engagement and reassessment in behavioral health specialty care and a select group of quality measures. These findings highlight areas in which the MHS delivers excellent care, as well as areas that should be targeted for quality improvement.

Acknowledgments

We gratefully acknowledge the support of our project sponsors, CDR Angela Williams (U.S. Public Health Service) and Kate McGraw, and staff at the Defense Centers of Excellence for Psychological Health and Traumatic Brain Injury. We appreciate the valuable insights we received from Daniel Kivlahan and Melony Sorbero. We addressed their constructive critiques as part of RAND's rigorous quality assurance process to improve the quality of this report. We also thank Lauren Skrabala and Tiffany Hruby for their assistance in preparation of this report, Dionne Barnes-Proby for her work to oversee human subjects and regulatory protocols and approvals for the project, and Carrie Farmer for her contribution to developing the plan for this work. Finally, we thank the DoD and VA clinical experts who provided input on portions of the medical record review tool, including LTC Christopher Ivany (Army), LTC Millard Brown (Army), LTC Wendi M. Waits (Army), CAPT John A. Ralph (Navy), CDR Michail Charissis (Navy), Jan E. Kemp (VA), and Dr. Steven Dobscha (VA). Their feedback helped to improve the review tool, in particular guiding the approach we used to capture suicide risk assessment and follow-up. Those who provided feedback are not responsible for the resulting final version of the tool or the results presented in this report.

Abbreviations

AHRQ	Agency for Healthcare Research and Quality
AUDIT	Alcohol Use Disorders Identification Test
AUDIT-C	Alcohol Use Disorders Identification Test–3-item screen
BH	behavioral health
BHDP	Behavioral Health Data Portal
CAPER	Comprehensive Ambulatory Professional Encounter Record
CBT	cognitive behavioral therapy
CDC-HRQOL	Centers for Disease Control and Prevention–Health Related Quality of Life
CMS	Centers for Medicare & Medicaid Services
CPG	clinical practice guideline
CPT	current procedural terminology
CPT	cognitive processing therapy
C-SSRS	Columbia Suicide Severity Rating Scale
DCoE	Defense Centers of Excellence for Psychological Health and Traumatic Brain Injury
DHA	Defense Health Agency
DMDC	Defense Manpower Data Center
DoD	U.S. Department of Defense
DSM-IV	Diagnostic and Statistical Manual of Mental Disorders, 4th ed.
DSM-5	Diagnostic and Statistical Manual of Mental Disorders, 5th ed.

EBT	evidence-based therapy
ED	emergency department
EQ-5D	European Quality of Life–5 Dimensions
EHR	electronic health record
E&M	evaluation and management
EMDR	eye movement desensitization and reprocessing
FY	fiscal year
GAD-7	Generalized Anxiety Disorder, 7-item
HA	Health Affairs
HEDIS	Healthcare Effectiveness Data and Information Set
HMO	Health Maintenance Organization
HRQOL	health-related quality of life
ICD-9-CM	International Classification of Diseases-9–Clinical Modification
IOM	Institute of Medicine
IPT	interpersonal psychotherapy
MDD	major depressive disorder
MDR	MHS Data Repository
MEPRS	Medical Expense & Performance Reporting System
MH	mental health
MHS	military health system
MRR	medical record review
MTF	military treatment facility
NCQA	National Committee for Quality Assurance
NQF	National Quality Forum
NTE	new treatment episode
OEF	Operation Enduring Freedom
OIF	Operation Iraqi Freedom

PABAK	prevalence and bias adjusted kappa
PCL	PTSD Checklist
PDTS	Pharmacy Data Transaction Service
PE	prolonged exposure
PH	psychological health
PHQ-2	Patient Health Questionnaire (two items)
PHQ-9	Patient Health Questionnaire (nine items)
PPO	Preferred Provider Organization
PST	problem-solving therapy
PTSD	posttraumatic stress disorder
RESPECT-Mil	Re-Engineering Systems of Primary Care Treatment in the Military
SD	standard deviation
SDS	Sheehan Disability Scale
SF-36	Short Form 36-Item Health Survey
SI	suicidal ideation
SIDR	Standard Inpatient Data Record
SIT	stress inoculation training
SNRI	serotonin and norepinephrine reuptake inhibitor
SSN	Social Security number
SSRI	selective serotonin reuptake inhibitor
SUD	substance use disorder
TBI	traumatic brain injury
TED-I	TRICARE Encounter Data–Institutional
TED-NI	TRICARE Encounter Data–Noninstitutional
TF-CBT	trauma-focused cognitive behavioral therapy
VHA	Veterans' Health Administration
VA	U.S. Department of Veterans Affairs

VM6   (V)irtual Storage Access Memory (M)ilitary Health System Data
                         Repository 200(6)

CHAPTER ONE

Introduction

Overview

In this chapter, we first provide an overview of a series of reports on quality care for posttraumatic stress disorder (PTSD) and depression delivered by the Military Health System (MHS), of which this is the third. We follow with the background and rationale for this report, information about PTSD and depression in service members, treatment of these conditions in the MHS, how quality of care is measured, related RAND projects conducted previously, and a list of the quality measures presented in this report.

This report represents the third in a series of RAND reports about assessing the quality of care for PTSD and depression in the MHS. At the request of the U.S. Department of Defense (DoD), the RAND Corporation initiated a project in 2012 to (1) provide a descriptive baseline assessment of the extent to which providers in the MHS implement care consistent with clinical practice guidelines (CPGs) for PTSD and depression, and (2) examine the relationship between guideline-concordant care and clinical outcomes for these conditions. This third and final report builds on prior RAND work in this area (Hepner et al., 2015; Hepner et al., 2016). Briefly, the first report (Hepner et al., 2015) presented a set of quality measures developed for measuring quality of care provided to active-component service members with PTSD and depression. The second report (Hepner et al., 2016), based on 2012–2013 administrative data, presented characteristics of active-component service members who received care for PTSD or depression from the MHS, along with an assessment of the quality of care provided for PTSD and depression using quality measures.

This report includes more quality measures and uses additional sources of data to provide a more comprehensive assessment of MHS care for PTSD and depression. We analyzed data from two new sources, medical record data and symptom questionnaire data. Medical record data, abstracted by trained raters from the outpatient electronic chart, capture more detailed clinical aspects of care not available from administrative data, such as assessment and follow-up of suicide risk, assessment for comorbid conditions (e.g., alcohol or drug use), and the psychotherapy approach used. We also obtained symptom questionnaire data for behavioral health conditions, which are available from a dedicated data collection system within MHS. Data from all sources were analyzed for the 2013–2014 time period, one year later than the time period used for the analyses in our previous report, which was 2012–2013 (Hepner et al., 2016). We describe the characteristics of active-component service members who received care for PTSD or depression from the MHS in 2013–2014 based on administrative data. We also assess the quality of care provided for PTSD and depression using quality measures based on all three data sources for 2013–2014. Finally, we explore the relationship between adherence to CPGs and symptom scores, limited to Army personnel who were seen in military treatment facility (MTF) behavioral health clinics, due to data availability.

Background and Rationale

Maintaining a healthy mission-ready force requires physical and psychological readiness of every service member. Achieving this goal requires that the MHS provides the highest quality care, including delivering effective prevention and treatment for both physical and psychological health (PH) conditions (DoD, 2014a). In the past decade, multiple reports have highlighted the need to provide high quality of care for PH conditions to military populations (Hoge, Auchterlonie, and Milliken, 2006; Tanielian and Jaycox, 2008). A series of Institute of Medicine (IOM) reports have repeatedly emphasized the strong need for the development of evidence-based quality measures, monitoring of the care provided to MHS beneficiaries for PH conditions, and implementation of systematic quality improvement efforts to improve outcomes. In a study of mental health counseling services under TRICARE, the IOM recommended a "comprehensive quality-management system for all mental health professionals" to monitor evidence-based practices and implement quality measures to assess the performance of mental health professionals (Institute of Medicine, 2010). A more recent IOM report focused on preventing psychological disorders in service members and their families and highlighted the need for evidence-based measures to evaluate interventions (Institute of Medicine, 2014a). Another recent IOM report (Institute of Medicine, 2014b) on the treatment of posttraumatic stress disorder (PTSD) in military and veteran populations emphasized that a "high-performing" system for managing PTSD requires quality measures and feedback to improve care. Such a system would entail the "systematic collection, analysis, and dissemination of data for assessing the quality of PTSD care."

Over recent years, the MHS has increased attention on assessing the quality of care delivered. A recent comprehensive review of the MHS (DoD, 2014c) found that on average, performance on many quality of care measures was similar to that of other health care systems, but significant variation in performance was observed across MTFs, resulting in many areas in need of improvement. In response to the report, former Defense Secretary Chuck Hagel (Secretary of Defense, 2014) called for MTFs

> "Quality, accountable health care is the most consequential benefit a grateful nation owes its Service members and their families. We are committed to improve and deliver on that commitment."
>
> —Jonathan Woodson, MD, then–Assistant Secretary of Defense for Health Affairs, June 2015 statement to the House Armed Services Committee (Woodson, 2015b)

that were low performers on quality and safety to create action plans for performance improvement. Further, he called for more transparency in providing patients, providers, and policymakers with information about quality and safety performance of the MHS. In January 2015, former Assistant Secretary of Defense for Health Affairs, Jonathan Woodson, announced the availability of information on quality and safety for individual MTFs on a newly created website, and plans for conducting meetings with beneficiary organizations and focus groups to solicit input on "how best to present and display these data" with the goal of launching the website with a "public outreach and communication campaign" (Woodson, 2015a). This website continues to evolve but provides information about accreditation of military hospitals and clinics, inpatient hospital quality measures, outpatient quality measures, and results of a beneficiary survey about access to health care and satisfaction with health care experiences.

Woodson highlighted DoD's commitment to transparency with his statement that DoD would "provide the public with 'all currently available aggregate statistical access, quality and safety information'," as directed by the Secretary of Defense (Woodson, 2016). Currently, only two measures related to PH care are included on this website. While these are commendable efforts, it is important for the MHS to continue to give increased attention to quality of PH care.

PTSD and Depression Among Service Members

Between 2001 and 2014, more than 2.6 million service members from the United States were deployed to Afghanistan in support of Operation Enduring Freedom (OEF) and to Iraq in support of Operation Iraqi Freedom (OIF) and Operation New Dawn (Institute of Medicine, 2014a). Rates of PTSD in active-duty service members who have served in OEF or OIF have been estimated at between 4 and 20 percent (Institute of Medicine, 2013). The rate of PTSD varies by service, with 4 percent of Air Force, 4.5 percent of Navy, 10 percent of Marines, and 13.5 percent of Army service members receiving a PTSD diagnosis (Institute of Medicine, 2014a). There are also differences in rates of PTSD diagnosis between male and female service members (9 percent versus 13 percent) and between whites and nonwhites (8.5 percent versus 11 percent).

A recent review (Ramchand et al., 2015) provided estimates of the prevalence of depression among veterans having served in OEF or OIF from studies published between 2009 and 2014, ranging from 1 percent of male veterans receiving care in Veterans Health Administration (VHA) facilities (Haskell et al., 2011) up to 60 percent of veterans referred to the New Jersey War Related Illness and Injury Study Center (WRIISC) (Helmer et al., 2009). This review (Ramchand et al., 2015) also reported an increased risk of depression for individuals who were female, white, not married, in the Army, enlisted, and lower in rank based on studies of current service members or veterans.

Care Provided to Service Members with PTSD and Depression

The MHS provides physical and PH care for active-component service members, National Guard and Reserve members, retirees, their families, survivors, and some former spouses worldwide. The health care resources of the Uniformed Services, known as direct care, are used to provide care through MTFs. At the end of fiscal year (FY) 2014, the MHS had about 9.5 million beneficiaries (DoD, 2014b). For FY 2015, the worldwide resources projected for the MHS are 151,785 employees, 55 hospitals (41 in the United States), 373 ambulatory care clinics (315 in the United States), and 264 dental clinics (210 in the United States) (DoD, 2014c). Direct care is supplemented by care provided outside of MTFs by civilian providers (i.e., health care professionals, institutions, pharmacies, and suppliers), known as purchased care. The civilian resources projected for use during FY 2015 include 550,194 primary care, behavioral health, and specialty care network providers, including 68,465 behavioral health network providers; 3,812 TRICARE network acute care hospitals; 1,757 behavioral health facilities; and 59,670 contracted retail pharmacies (DoD, 2015).

Programs and services for prevention, diagnosis, and treatment of psychological health conditions, including PTSD and depression, are available to all service members in DoD (Institute of Medicine, 2014a). Although not specific to PTSD and depression, prevention programs developed by each branch of the service include training and services meant to "foster mental resilience, preserve mission readiness, and mitigate adverse consequences of exposure to stress" (Institute of Medicine, 2014a). Before deployment, each service member is screened for previous psychological health care. Service members returning from deployment are screened for symptoms of PTSD and depression at 30 days and three to six months. Referral for further care is based on results of the screening. Individuals with symptoms of PTSD or depression are often treated on an outpatient basis through mental health clinics, primary care settings by primary care practitioners and mental health professionals, and programs targeting PTSD and/or depression. These programs reside in the service branches, and in TRICARE contract programs. Other treatment options include intensive outpatient programs that utilize psychotherapy and pharmacotherapy, in addition to complementary therapies (e.g., acupuncture, yoga, meditation). Inpatient treatment for PTSD and depression is available in MTFs as direct care and from other providers and facilities through purchased care.

Measuring the Quality of Health Care

Quality measures provide a way to measure how well health care is being delivered. Quality measures are applied by operationalizing aspects of care recommended by the clinical practice guidelines (CPGs) using data sources such as administrative data, medical records, clinical registries, and patient surveys. Such measures provide information about the health care system and highlight areas in which providers can take action to make health care safer and reduce health disparities (National Quality Forum [NQF], 2017a and 2017b). Quality measures incorporate operationally defined numerators and denominators, and scores are typically presented as the percentage of eligible patients who received the recommended care (e.g., percentage of PTSD patients screened for co-occurring depression). According to the Agency for Healthcare Research and Quality (Agency for Healthcare Research and Quality, undated), quality measures are generally used by organizations for quality improvement, accountability, and research. Measuring adherence to CPGs using quality measures can establish a baseline assessment of care against which future improvements can be compared, identify potential areas for quality improvement, and provide support for developing an infrastructure to continuously improve the quality of PH care provided to patients.

Delivering high-quality health care is a priority of the MHS. Health Affairs (HA) Policy 02-016 (Health Affairs, 2002) laid out the fundamentals of the MHS quality of health care system. A comprehensive review of access to care, quality of care, and patient safety in the MHS highlighted movement toward a "high-reliability health system" (DoD, 2014c). High-priority goals for improving performance were stated to be "harm prevention and quality improvement" supported by "better analytics, greater clarity in policy, and aligned training and education programs" (DoD, 2014c). CPGs set standards for appropriate care and represent expert consensus, after systematic review of relevant literature, on how a condition should be diagnosed and treated. For example, the VA and DoD have published CPGs for the management of major depressive disorder (MDD) (VA and DoD 2009) and posttraumatic stress (VA and DoD, 2010), and these guidelines describe evidence-based processes of care. It should be noted that the PTSD CPG is currently in the process of being updated, and an updated version of the MDD CPG was recently published (VA and DoD, 2016).

Other than our previous report (Hepner et al., 2016), little is known about the level of adherence to the recommendations of CPGs for much of the care for psychological health conditions in the MHS. Furthermore, there is currently no MHS-wide system in place to routinely assess the quality of care provided for PTSD and depression or to understand whether the care is having a positive effect on outcomes.

Previous RAND Projects on Assessing Quality of PH Care

RAND has conducted prior work, also funded by DCoE, which provides an essential foundation for the work presented in this report. The two reports are briefly described below.

Candidate Quality Measures Report (Hepner et al., 2015): We developed a conceptual framework for assessing the quality of care for PH conditions and identified candidate quality measures for monitoring, assessing, and improving care for PTSD and MDD (Hepner et al., 2015). The two-dimensional framework was used to classify 58 measures according to measure type (structure, process, outcome, patient experience, and resource use) and continuum of care domain (prevention, screening, assessment, treatment, and integration). We used a systematic expert consensus process to select measures based on their validity, importance to PH, feasibility of implementation within MHS, and NQF endorsement status. Technical specifications, which extensively detail the method for calculating each measure score, were developed or adapted for each of the PTSD and depression measures.

Phase I Report (Hepner et al., 2016): We evaluated the quality of PTSD and depression care for active-component service members using 12 (six for each condition) of the originally identified set of quality measures. These measures, derived from administrative data, assess adequate medication trial and management, receipt of any psychotherapy, receipt of minimal number of psychotherapy or medication management visits, timely follow-up after hospitalization, and utilization of inpatient care. The study found the quality of MHS PTSD and depression care to be excellent in some areas, and in need of improvement in others. For example, the MHS demonstrated high percentages with timely follow-up after discharge from a psychiatric hospitalization (86 percent received follow-up within seven days of discharge). However, a third of PTSD cohort patients and less than a quarter of those in the depression cohort received adequate care (defined as four psychotherapy visits or two medication management visits) within the first eight weeks of a new treatment episode. Several policy recommendations were offered based on these findings, including the need to improve the quality of care for PH health conditions delivered by the MHS, and the need to establish an enterprise-wide performance measurement system to track key quality measures for PH care.

PTSD and Depression Quality of Care

PTSD and Depression Quality Measures

In this report, we assess the quality of outpatient care delivered using 30 quality measures (15 each for PTSD and depression). These measures include both process measures (24 measures) and outcome measures (six measures). In the continuum of care, they include assessment measures (eight measures) and treatment measures (22 measures). For each of the two conditions, five measures are based on administrative data, seven are based on data collected from medical records, and three measures are based on symptom questionnaire data. These measures are listed in Table 1.1, and measure results are described in Chapters Four and Five. Detailed technical specifications are provided in Appendixes A and B[1] for PTSD and depression measures, respectively.

Table 1.1
PTSD and Depression Quality Measures

Measure No.	PTSD	Depression
	Assessment	
A1	Percentage of PTSD patients with a new treatment episode with assessment of symptoms with PCL within 30 days	Percentage of depression patients with a new treatment episode with assessment of symptoms with PHQ-9 within 30 days
A2	Percentage of PTSD patients with a new treatment episode assessed for depression within 30 days	Percentage of depression patients with a new treatment episode assessed for manic/hypomanic behaviors within 30 days
A3	Percentage of PTSD patients with a new treatment episode assessed for suicide risk at same visit	Percentage of depression patients with a new treatment episode assessed for suicide risk at same visit[a]
A4	Percentage of PTSD patients with a new treatment episode assessed for recent substance use within 30 days	Percentage of depression patients with a new treatment episode assessed for recent substance use within 30 days
	Treatment	
T1	Percentage of PTSD patients with symptom assessment with PCL during 4-month measurement period	Percentage of depression patients with symptom assessment with PHQ-9 during 4-month measurement period[a]
T3	Percentage of patient contacts of PTSD patients with SI with appropriate follow-up (PTSD-T3)	Percentage of patient contacts of depression patients with SI with appropriate follow-up (Depression-T3)
T5	Percentage of PTSD patients with a newly prescribed SSRI/SNRI with an adequate trial (≥60 days)	Percentage of depression patients with a newly prescribed antidepressant with a trial of 12 weeks (T5a) or 6 months (T5b)[a]
T6	Percentage of PTSD patients newly prescribed an SSRI/SNRI with follow-up visit within 30 days	Percentage of depression patients newly prescribed an antidepressant with follow-up visit within 30 days

---

[1]   Available online with this report: http://www.rand.org/pubs/research_reports/RR1542.html.

Table 1.1—Continued

Measure No.	PTSD	Depression
T7	Percentage of PTSD patients who receive evidence-based psychotherapy for PTSD	Percentage of depression patients who receive evidence-based psychotherapy for depression
T8	Percentage of PTSD patients with a new treatment episode who received any psychotherapy within the first 4 months	Percentage of depression patients with a new treatment episode who received any psychotherapy within the first 4 months
T9	Percentage of PTSD patients with a new treatment episode with 4 psychotherapy visits or 2 evaluation and management visits in the first 8 weeks	Percentage of depression patients with a new treatment episode with 4 psychotherapy visits or 2 evaluation and management visits in the first 8 weeks
T10	Percentage of PTSD patients (PCL score >43) with response to treatment (5-point reduction in PCL score) at 6 months	Percentage of depression patients (PHQ-9 score >9) with response to treatment (50% reduction in PHQ-9 score) at 6 months[a]
T12	Percentage of PTSD patients (PCL score >43) in PTSD-symptom remission (PCL score <28) at 6 months	Percentage of depression patients (PHQ-9 score >9) in depression-symptom remission (PHQ-9 score<5) at 6 months[a]
T14	Percentage of PTSD patients with a new treatment episode with improvement in functional status at 6 months	Percentage of depression patients with a new treatment episode with improvement in functional status at 6 months
T15	Percentage of psychiatric inpatient hospital discharges of patients with PTSD with follow-up in 7 days (T15a) or 30 days (T15b)[a]	Percentage of psychiatric inpatient hospital discharges of patients with depression with follow-up in 7 days (T15a) or 30 days (T15b)[a]

NOTE: PCL = PTSD Checklist; PHQ-9 = Patient Health Questionnaire, 9-item; SSRI = selective serotonin reuptake inhibitor; SNRI = serotonin and norepinephrine reuptake inhibitor.

[a] NQF-endorsed measure.

Clinical Outcomes Related to PTSD and Depression

In this report, we examine the association between the quality of care received and clinical outcomes using multivariate analyses among service members with PTSD or depression. Quality of care is based on administrative data–based quality measures (four each for PTSD and depression) and clinical outcomes on symptom question-naires from service members through behavioral health clinics at MTFs. We also describe the patterns of symptom questionnaire completion overall and by month at MTFs and how symptom scores change over time among service members with PTSD or depression in 2013–2014.

Organization of This Report

This report provides a description of the characteristics of active-component service members diagnosed with PTSD or depression in the MHS in January through June of 2013. We also assessed the quality of care provided for PTSD and depression using quality measures based on administrative data, medical record data, and data from symptom questionnaires. In analyses of administrative data, we included care delivered in MTFs as direct care and through other providers and facilities as purchased care. Our analyses included medical record data for direct care only, and symptom questionnaire data for Army personnel receiving mental health specialty care in the direct care system. Understanding the current status of care is an important step toward future efforts to improve care, including the development of an ongoing quality monitoring process.

Chapter Two describes the data sources and methods used to operationalize and apply the PTSD and depression quality measures using three sources of data: administrative data, medical record data, and symptom questionnaire data. The methods used to analyze the characteristics of those in the two cohorts and the quality measures are also described. **Chapter Three** includes results describing the characteristics of the service members with a PTSD or depression diagnosis and their utilization of health care services in the MHS in 2013–2014. **Chapters Four and Five** present results on the quality of care provided for **PTSD** and **depression**, respectively. **Chapter Six** examines the use of symptom questionnaires and the relationship between quality of care and symptom scores for Army personnel in the PTSD and depression cohorts who received mental health specialty care. **Chapter Seven** summarizes the main findings of the report and provides policy implications that follow from the findings.

A series of online appendixes are also available with this report: www.rand.org/pubs/research_reports/RR1542.html. **Appendixes A and B** contain technical specifications for the PTSD and depression quality measures, respectively. **Appendix C** describes the methods used for the medical record review sample and data collection. **Appendix D** presents results on variation in measure scores on the administrative data–based quality measures by member and service-related characteristics for PTSD and depression. **Appendix E** presents detailed results for the multivariable logistic and linear regression models, which were run to analyze the PCL scores for PTSD and the PHQ-9 scores for depression.

CHAPTER TWO

Methods

Overview

In this chapter, we describe the methods used to conduct the analyses presented in this report. We describe data sources used for the analyses, along with a brief description of how we processed each of the three types of data available to us:

1. For the **administrative data** analyses, we describe how we identified the PTSD and depression cohorts of active-component service members, the methods for the descriptive analyses, and the analyses to examine the quality measure results and explore variations in care.
2. For the analyses of **medical record data**, we describe how we identified a smaller sample for medical record review from the PTSD and depression cohorts, the development of a data collection tool, abstraction of medical record data, and the analyses to examine the quality measure results.
3. For the analyses of **symptom questionnaire data**, we describe how the data were collected, how frequently service members in the PTSD and depression cohorts complete the symptom questionnaires, what analyses (both quality measure score results and multivariate regression) were performed based on these data, and what methods were used for each application.

Table 2.1 provides a list of data files used in the analyses. The detailed technical specifications for the application of the quality measures, rationale for their use (from the literature and clinical practice guidelines), and feasibility of use can be found in Appendixes A and B for PTSD and depression, respectively.[1] All study methods were approved by the RAND Human Subjects Protection Committee, as well as by the U.S. Army Medical Research and Materiel Command's Human Research Protection Office.

---

[1] Appendixes for this report are available online: http://www.rand.org/pubs/research_reports/RR1542.html.

Table 2.1
Content of Data Files Used in Analyses

Content	Data Files
Administrative Data	
Outpatient services delivered within MTFs (direct care)	Comprehensive Ambulatory Professional Encounter Record (CAPER)
Inpatient services delivered within MTFs (direct care)	Standard Inpatient Data Record (SIDR)
Provider services delivered outside of MTFs (purchased care)	TRICARE Encounter Data–Noninstitutional (TED-NI)
Facility services delivered outside of MTFs (purchased care)	TRICARE Encounter Data–Institutional (TED-I)
TRICARE eligibility and enrollment	VM6 Beneficiary Level
TRICARE eligibility/active-duty status	Active-Duty Master File
Dispensed medication	Pharmacy Data Transaction Services (PDTS)
Service characteristics	Defense Manpower Data Center (DMDC)
Deployment history (September 2001 through March 2015)	Contingency Tracking System–Deployments
Medical Record Data	
Medical record of outpatient care delivered within MTFs (direct care)	AHLTA
Symptom Questionnaire Data	
Patient responses to symptom questionnaires (e.g., PCL, PHQ-9)	Behavioral Health Data Portal (BHDP)

NOTE: MTF = military treatment facility.

Administrative Data

We used several sources of MHS administrative data to identify the eligible diagnostic cohorts, describe their characteristics, construct many of the quality measures, and conduct many of the analyses described in this report. While a previous RAND report focused on care provided from January 2012 through June 2013 (Hepner et al., 2016), the administrative data analyzed for this report include care provided to active-component service members over an 18-month period from January 1, 2013, through June 30, 2014. We focused on active-component service members to increase the likelihood that the care they received was provided or paid for by the MHS, rather than other sources of health care. Members of the National Guard and Reserve components, retirees, and family members were not included in these analyses. Active-component service members can obtain health care provided by the Military Health System in two ways: care provided in MTFs, which is called direct care, and care provided by civilian providers and paid for by TRICARE, which is called purchased care. We used extract files of administrative data for these two types of care created by the Defense Health Agency (DHA) from the MHS Data Repository (MDR). These files contain records on all inpatient and outpatient health care encounters for TRICARE beneficiaries paid (fully or partially) by TRICARE (Table 2.1). We included all inpatient and outpatient health care encounters for direct care and purchased care. All records for an individual were de-duplicated and linked.[2]

Processing Inpatient and Outpatient Encounter Data

Preparing encounter data for use in calculating the quality measures entailed extensive processing of direct care inpatient and outpatient stay records (the SIDR and CAPER files) and of purchased care provider and facility records (the TED-NI and TED-I files) to ensure that encounters (i.e., outpatient visits, inpatient stays) were accurately counted. Here we provide a brief overview of the decisions made in processing these data. The detailed steps in this process, including variable names and codes, are documented in the appendix of the Phase I report of this study (Hepner et al., 2016).

The first step of processing the acute care inpatient encounter data was developing a definition of an encounter and applying rules to operationalize the definition. To avoid double-counting, we eliminated duplicate records for the same inpatient stay. Because our analysis included only inpatient care provided in acute care facilities, all nonacute care (i.e., rehabilitation care, residential/extended care, skilled nursing facility care, and home care) was excluded from the file of acute inpatient stays. The rules were applied to records in both the direct care inpatient file (i.e., SIDR) and the purchased care facility file (i.e., TED-I).

Similar rules were applied to outpatient encounters. Multiple lines of data with the same provider specialty on the same date were counted as a single outpatient visit for that specialty. Multiple records for the emergency department or ambulatory surgery on the same date were counted as a single outpatient visit, regardless of the number of providers or specialties involved. Other than emergency department or ambulatory surgery, encounter records on the same day with providers in different specialties (other than radiology) were counted as separate outpatient visits. Encounter records with providers who generally provide ancillary services, such as general duty nurses and corpsmen,,were not counted as separate outpatient visits. These rules were applied to records in both the direct care outpatient file (i.e., CAPER) and the purchased care provider and facility files (i.e., TED-NI and TED-I).

---

[2]   Pharmacy Data Transaction Service (PDTS) files included only the scrambled Social Security number (SSN) of the plan sponsor. It was expected that the majority of the sponsors were the active-component members. To identify nonsponsor files, cross checks between the PDTS and the Virtual Storage Access Memory Military Health System Data Repository 2006 (VM6) Beneficiary Level files were made to compare age and gender. Those cases that were not matches to gender or age category (one age-category change to the next level during the 12-month measurement period was allowed) were dropped from the analyses.

Identification of Service Members in PTSD and Depression Cohorts
To describe and evaluate care for PTSD and depression, we identified a cohort of service members who received care coded with at least one PTSD or depression diagnosis. We selected eligibility criteria aimed at identifying cohorts of patients diagnosed with PTSD or depression who were likely to receive all or the majority of their care from the MHS. Figure 2.1 shows the cohort selection process with the eligibility criteria used to identify each diagnostic cohort. The eligibility criteria for selecting these diagnostic cohorts consisted of all of the following:

Active-Component Service Members—The patient must have been an active-component service member during the entire 12-month observation period.

Received Care for PTSD or Depression—Service members could enter the PTSD or depression cohort if they had at least one outpatient visit or inpatient stay (direct or purchased care) with a PTSD or depression diagnosis

Figure 2.1
Eligibility Criteria for Cohort Entry

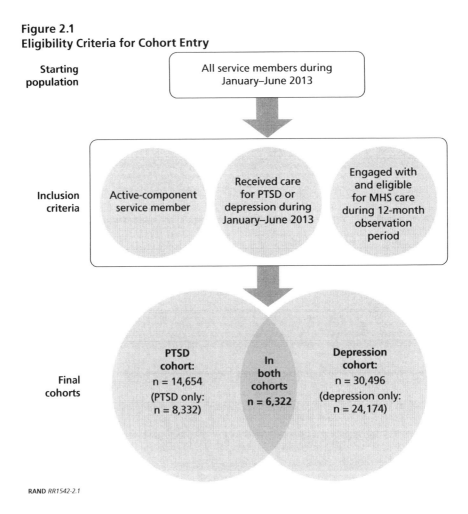

(primary or secondary) during January through June 2013, as documented in administrative data.

Engaged with and Eligible for MHS Care—Service members were eligible for a cohort if they had received a minimum of one inpatient stay or two out-patient visits for any diagnosis (i.e., related or unrelated to PTSD or depression) within the MHS (either direct or purchased care) during the 12-month observation period following the index visit. This minimal engagement in MHS care was used to increase the likelihood that the MHS was the member's primary source of health care. In addition, service members must have been eligible for TRICARE benefits during the entire 12-month observation period. Members who deployed or separated from the service during the 12-month period were excluded.

Using these criteria, we identified 14,654 service members for the 2013–2014 PTSD cohort and 30,496 for the 2013–2014 depression cohort. The two cohorts were not mutually exclusive, so it was possible for a service member to be in both the PTSD and depression cohorts based on diagnoses at the time of cohort entry. A total of 6,322 service members were in both cohorts, representing 43.1 percent of the PTSD cohort and 20.7 percent of the depression cohort. Therefore, the two cohorts together represent a total of 38,828 unique service members. While we considered presenting results separately for the subgroups included in both cohorts, we believe that the focus only on the comorbidity between PTSD and depression would ignore other relevant comorbidities and would be an artifact of the two diagnoses selected for this work. Figure 2.2

Figure 2.2
Timing of Cohort Entry and Computation of 12-month Observation Period

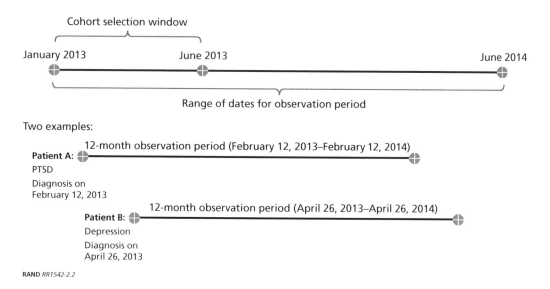

shows the period during which service members could enter a cohort (cohort selection window) and the period during which we assessed their care (observation period).

Cohort Considerations

We carefully considered how to identify each cohort. One key decision was the requirement of only one PTSD or depression diagnosis for cohort entry.[3] We opted to include patients with only one diagnosis because it was essential to not exclude patients with an accurate PTSD or depression diagnosis who did not receive indicated follow-up care. This approach may include a subset of patients whose diagnosis was inaccurate or changed in a subsequent visit. However, our analysis of the cohorts identified in this way revealed that 87 percent of the PTSD cohort and 81 percent of the depression cohort had two or more encounters associated with a cohort diagnosis (primary or secondary) during their 12-month observation period. We also conducted a sensitivity analysis to compare scores for quality measures that require a single PTSD (or depression) diagnosis (original specifications) to measure scores based on a denominator limited to service members with at least two PTSD (or depression) diagnoses (restricted specification). The results of these analyses indicated that requiring two diagnoses had little impact on the measure scores (see Chapters Four and Five).

When defining the depression cohort, we also chose to include patients with diagnosis codes other than just those for MDD. We included codes that have been used for identifying the denominators for NQF-endorsed depression measures, including dysthymia and other depressive disorders (e.g., ICD-9 codes 300.4, 311). We also retained a broader definition due to the concern that ICD-9 code 311 has been shown to be used frequently by providers as a "catch all" to code MDD (National Quality Forum, 2014b). An analysis of our depression cohort revealed that 37 percent had an MDD diagnosis code at some point during the observation year. Another 51 percent of the cohort without an MDD diagnosis had a diagnosis of depressive disorder, not otherwise specified (ICD-9 code 311). We acknowledge that the relevant CPG specifically targets patients with MDD rather than just any depression, and therefore, some measures reported here will require further validation. However, the newly updated CPG for MDD does recommend considering the principles in the updated guideline when treating other depressive disorders and, in particular, unspecified depressive disorders (VA and DoD, 2016).

Finally, we selected eligibility criteria to increase the likelihood that service members included in the cohorts were likely to receive their care from the MHS. For example, we excluded service members who separated or were deployed during their 12-month observation period. It is notable that 41 percent were excluded from the PTSD cohort and 35 percent were excluded from the depression cohort because of fail-

---

[3]   ICD-9 code for PTSD: 309.81; ICD-9 codes for depression: 296.20–296.26, 296.30–296.36, 293.83, 296.90, 296.99, 298.0, 300.4, 309.1, and 311.

ure to meet eligibility requirements, suggesting that they separated from the military during their observation year. This is a sizable population of particular interest that will be important to study further. The proportion excluded from each cohort due to deployment was minimal (3 percent for PTSD; 5 percent for depression).

Administrative Data Quality Measures

We developed or adapted technical specifications for a total of ten administrative data measures (five each for PTSD and for depression); these ten measures are listed in Table 2.2.[4] The set of five administrative data measures assess care described in the VA/DoD CPGs, including adequate medication trial (T5) and medication management (T6), receipt of any psychotherapy (T8), receipt of a minimum number of visits associated with a first-line treatment (either psychotherapy or medication management) (T9), and follow-up after psychiatric hospitalization (T15). Among these treatment process measures, some focus on care provided to a subset of patients in a "new treatment episode"

Table 2.2
PTSD and Depression Quality Measures Using Administrative Data

Measure No.	PTSD	Depression
	Treatment	
T5	Percentage of PTSD patients with a newly prescribed SSRI/SNRI with an adequate trial of (≥ 60 days)	Percentage of depression patients with a newly prescribed antidepressant with a trial of 12 weeks (T5a) or 6 months (T5b)[a]
T6	Percentage of PTSD patients newly prescribed an SSRI/SNRI with follow-up visit within 30 days	Percentage of depression patients newly prescribed an antidepressant with follow-up visit within 30 days
T8	Percentage of PTSD patients with a new treatment episode who received any psychotherapy within the first 4 months	Percentage of depression patients with a new treatment episode who received any psychotherapy within the first 4 months
T9	Percentage of PTSD patients with a new treatment episode with 4 psychotherapy visits or 2 evaluation and management visits within the first 8 weeks	Percentage of depression patients with a new treatment episode with 4 psychotherapy visits or 2 evaluation and management visits within the first 8 weeks
T15	Percentage of psychiatric inpatient hospital discharges of patients with PTSD with follow-up in 7 days (T15a) or 30 days (T15b)[a]	Percentage of psychiatric inpatient hospital discharges of patients with depression with follow-up in 7 days (T15a) or 30 days (T15b)[a]

[a] NQF-endorsed measure.

---

[4]   The Phase I report included 12 administrative data measures and this report includes ten administrative data measures. The two measures representing the percentage of psychiatric discharges (RU1) for the PTSD and depression cohorts were not included in this report as quality measures because they focus on resource use rather than quality of care for PTSD or depression. However, information on inpatient utilization is presented in Table 3.5 (Chapter Three).

(NTE). These are patients who receive care for the cohort diagnosis (i.e., PTSD or depression) after a period of at least six months without any care for that diagnosis (a "clean period"), either in outpatient or inpatient care or by treatment with a condition-specific medication. The complete technical specifications for all administrative data measures are provided in Appendixes A and B for PTSD and depression, respectively.[5]

Strengths and Limitations of Using Administrative Data to Assess Care for PTSD and Depression

The administrative data used for our analyses are comprehensive, including data on every visit delivered through direct care (i.e., at MTFs) and purchased care (i.e., paid for by TRICARE, the health insurance provided to active-duty service members, and delivered through contracted providers). No other data source (e.g., medical record review, patient survey, provider survey) allows for such a comprehensive examination of all care provided by the MHS. However, administrative data do have some limitations. First, identification of individuals eligible for the PTSD and depression cohorts was based on diagnosis codes assigned by the practitioner and is subject to error. A service member without one of these conditions may have been assigned a PTSD or depression code in error (or to indicate diagnosis as a "rule out" or tentative diagnosis). Conversely, a service member with one of these conditions may not have been assigned a PTSD or depression code. Second, administrative data do not capture detailed aspects of treatment, such as medication refusals or contraindications typically documented only within the medical record; these details may be important in that they may justify departures from standard care. Third, routine outcome monitoring of symptoms is typically absent from administrative data, so tracking the clinical course and response to treatment for a particular patient is usually not possible. For these reasons, our quality measures based on medical record data and symptom question-naire data supply important information about quality of care. We describe these data sources in the next sections.

Medical Record Review Data

Medical record review was conducted on a stratified, random sample of service members from the PTSD and depression cohorts, limiting the sample to service members who received only direct care during the observation period. This limitation was based on the fact that medical records documenting purchased care were not accessible for abstraction. The source of medical record data was AHLTA, the electronic health record

---

[5]   For each measure in the study, the technical specifications include the following elements: measure title, measure statement, numerator, denominator, measure type, care setting, numerator specifications, denominator specifications, measure source, the rationale for including the measure, and the feasibility of measuring performance from existing data.

used by the MTFs to document outpatient care. Therefore, service members who may have had a change in service location (i.e., permanent change of station [PCS]) were still included in the sample. Inpatient care records were not accessed because the medical record–based measures focus only on outpatient care. Medical record review incorporated a hybrid methodology where administrative data were used, where applicable, to identify service members within the MRR sample with characteristics relevant to quality measure eligibility.

Selection of the Medical Record Review Sample

Figure 2.3 provides an overview of the selection of the MRR sample. Beginning with the PTSD and depression cohorts (as identified in Figure 2.2), the study population was further restricted to the 16,173 service members in the Army, Air Force, Marine Corps, and Navy[6,7] who received only direct care during their observation year (since we had access to medical records only from direct care). For purposes of yielding two distinct MRR samples for PTSD and depression, we randomly assigned each of the 1,616 service members with both PTSD and depression to either the PTSD or the depression cohort,[8] resulting in 4,514 and 11,659 service members, respectively, eligible for being randomly sampled for the MRR (Figure 2.3). From each of these groups, we drew a random sample of 400 service members from each of the PTSD and depression cohorts. Service members with an NTE on the first day of cohort entry were oversampled to ensure the final sample would include a sufficient number of service members eligible for the ten of the 14 MRR quality indicators focusing on NTEs.[9] The cohort sample size of 400 allows for the precision, or half-width of a 95 percent confidence interval, of a measure score estimate for an NTE-focused quality indicator or a quality indicator applying to the full cohort to be at most 6.6 percentage points.[10] Thus, the sample size is not large enough to make precise estimates by service branch, region, or service member characteristics, as we are able to do with the administrative data quality measures. The sample was also stratified to ensure that service members were sam-

---

[6]   Coast Guard service members were not sampled, since their relatively small proportion in the service member population would not allow for a sufficient number of them to be sampled to yield Coast Guard–specific estimates.

[7]   Those with missing region are excluded from the sampled population.

[8]   The probability of random assignment to the PTSD cohort is higher (0.70 versus 0.30) since the proportion of the cohort with both PTSD and depression is higher for the PTSD (32 percent) than the depression cohort (12 percent).

[9]   NTEs were limited to those that occurred on Day 1 of cohort entry (representing 96 and 97 percent of the total NTEs for PTSD and depression, respectively) to maximize the length of the observation period. Those with NTEs only occurring after Day 1 of cohort entry (e.g., a patient could have entered the cohort in ongoing treatment and then had a three-month clean period with no treatment, followed by receiving treatment again) were not sampled.

[10]   The precision is lowest for measure score estimates of 50 percent, but could be as low as 2.6 percent for a measure score estimate of 5 percent.

Figure 2.3
Process for Drawing the MRR Sample

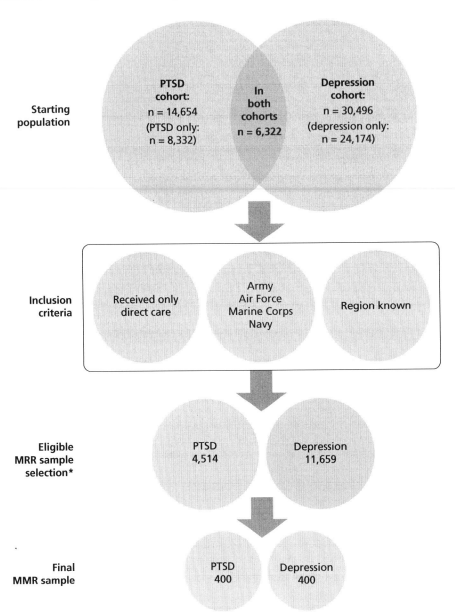

NOTE: * To yield two distinct MRR samples for PTSD and depression, the 1,616 with both conditions were randomly assigned to either PTSD (70 percent) or depression (30 percent). More service members were assigned to PTSD because a larger proportion of the PTSD cohort has both conditions (33 percent) versus the depression cohort (13 percent).

RAND RR1542-2.3

pled by branch, region, and by having both PTSD and depression versus having one of these conditions. Sampling weights for estimating the measure scores of the NTE and all-cohort quality measures were applied to account for the stratified sampling plan. See Appendix C for a detailed description of the MRR sampling methodology.

Medical Record Review Methods

A contracted vendor with prior experience remotely accessing and abstracting mental health records within the military's outpatient electronic health record system, AHLTA, conducted the medical record review. We worked with the vendor to create an online abstraction tool that would guide abstractors in the data collection and allow for direct data entry. We trained abstractors in the use of the tool, evaluated their level of performance prior to initiating abstraction, and created an ongoing system to address questions and issues that arose during data collection. During data collection it was noted that the time needed to abstract a record exceeded time and budget constraints, necessitating a reduction in the amount of data collected. As a result, six quality measures (three each for PTSD and depression) initially in the MRR measure set were applied using symptom questionnaire data instead. MRR data collection was completed over a period of three months. Double abstractions were performed on a random sample of patients to evaluate interrater reliability. A more detailed description of the medical record review methods can be found in Appendix C. The medical record abstraction tool used to collect these data is available on request from the authors.

Medical Record Quality Measures

A total of 14 quality measures (seven each for PTSD and depression) rely on data abstracted from the medical record (Table 2.3). For each condition, four measures (A1–A4) focus on assessment, and the remaining measures focus on treatment. Most of the measures address processes of care, and one (T14) is an outcome measure. The majority of the measures used administrative data to identify the service members potentially eligible for each measure (e.g., had a new treatment episode), while information about the receipt of the recommended care was derived from the medical record. One measure (T3) was implemented entirely from medical record data. The complete technical specifications for all medical record measures are provided in Appendixes A and B for PTSD and depression, respectively.[11]

---

[11] For each measure in the study, the technical specifications include the following elements: measure title, measure statement, numerator, denominator, measure type, care setting, numerator specifications, denominator specifications, measure source, the rationale for including the measure, and the feasibility of measuring performance from existing data. These are provided in Appendixes A and B for PTSD and depression, respectively.

Table 2.3
PTSD and Depression Quality Measures Using Medical Record Data[a]

Measure No.	PTSD	Depression
Assessment		
A1	Percentage of PTSD patients with a new treatment episode assessed with the PCL within 30 days	Percentage of depression patients with a new treatment episode assessed with the PHQ-9 within 30 days
A2	Percentage of PTSD patients with a new treatment episode assessed for depression within 30 days	Percentage of depression patients with a new treatment episode assessed for manic/hypomanic behaviors within 30 days
A3	Percentage of PTSD patients with a new treatment episode assessed for suicide risk at same visit	Percentage of depression patients with a new treatment episode assessed for suicide risk at same visit[b]
A4	Percentage of PTSD patients with a new treatment episode assessed for recent substance use within 30 days	Percentage of depression patients with a new treatment episode assessed for recent substance use within 30 days
Treatment		
T3	Percentage of PTSD patient contacts with suicidal ideation with appropriate follow-up at same visit	Percentage of depression patient contacts with suicidal ideation with appropriate follow-up at same visit
T7	Percentage of PTSD patients who receive evidence-based psychotherapy for PTSD	Percentage of depression patients who receive evidence-based psychotherapy for depression
T14	Percentage of PTSD patients with a new treatment episode with improvement in functional status at 6 months	Percentage of depression patients with a new treatment episode with improvement in functional status at 6 months

[a] During the study, time and budget constraints resulted in a reduction in scope of the medical record abstraction. As a result, six measures (PTSD T1, T10, and T12 and Depression T1, T10, and T12) intended to be assessed with MRR data were assessed using symptom questionnaire data instead.

[b] NQF-endorsed measure for major depressive disorder.

Strengths and Limitations of Medical Record Review Data

The application of medical record review–based quality measures allowed us to collect care information not typically available through other data sources, such as administrative data. For example, using medical record review data, we are able to assess whether a provider delivered appropriate follow-up after identifying suicidal ideation and whether psychotherapy delivered was evidence-based. There were some limitations associated with the medical record review data. First, the MRR sample was limited to service members who received direct care only during their observation period. While this was necessary based on the nonavailability of purchased care records, we were unable to apply the MRR quality measures to the population of those who received purchased care alone or in combination with direct care. Relatedly, the medical record review did not capture care not paid for by TRICARE. The focus on service members who received direct care only resulted in some differences between the MRR samples and the full cohorts. For example, a larger portion of each cohort had both PTSD and depression (43 percent and 21 percent for the PTSD and depression cohorts, respectively) in the administrative data (Figure 2.1). Analogous percentages for the population eligible for the MRR, restricted to those receiving direct care only, were 33 percent and 13 percent, respectively, indicating less comorbidity in the MRR samples versus the full cohorts. Generalizability of the MRR findings to the full cohorts is limited by this difference. In addition, due to the time-intensive process to collect medical record data, we were limited to a sample, rather than the full population available in administrative data. Therefore, sample sizes for some quality measures are small and do not allow for evaluation of variability in care as we were able to do for the administrative data measures. Further, we note that although we are able to assess more detailed aspects of care by reviewing the medical record, there can be errors in documentation (e.g., inadequate or inaccurate documentation), including omission of documentation of care provided. Finally, some variables abstracted from the medical record are complex. In particular, assessing whether the psychotherapy delivered was evidence based was particularly challenging. A recent Institute of Medicine report (2015) highlighted the need for additional work to accurately assess the quality of psychosocial interventions, including psychotherapy. Assessing whether a patient received appropriate follow-up given his or her level of severity of suicidal risk was also quite difficult, as the most recent clinical practice guidelines for suicide VA and DoD, 2013) suggest categorizing patients by risk as a chief guide to appropriate follow-up. Our work is one of the first efforts to assess whether care aligned with these guidelines.

Medical record abstraction is a time-intensive process further burdened by AHLTA-related operational issues. The mechanics of opening and closing individual encounters within AHLTA contributed significantly to the average abstractor data collection time per record. Service members in the MRR sample had medical record notes associated with several outpatient visits during the observation period, pushing the average abstraction time over budgetary limitations. For example, the median number of outpatient visits was 24 (range 1 to 160) for PTSD patients in the sample and 21.5 (range 1 to 246) for depression patients. This factor led to a reduction in the amount of data collected and, therefore, a reduction in the number of quality measures that could be computed from the medical record data.

Symptom Questionnaire Data

Symptom scores for behavioral health conditions, based on questionnaires such as the PTSD Checklist (PCL) for PTSD and the Patient Health Questionnaire-9 (PHQ-9) for depression, are available from a dedicated data collection system within MHS. The system, known as the Behavioral Health Data Portal (BHDP), has been in operation since September 2013 in all of Army's behavioral health clinics. In September 2013, former Assistant Secretary of Defense (Health Affairs) mandated "measurement and documentation of clinical outcomes in mental health treatment [in all BH clinics] in Military Treatment Facilities (MTFs)" (Woodson, 2013). On August 26, 2014, President Obama issued executive actions related to mental health care in VA and DoD that mandated access to the BHDP for all providers, patients, and clinical leaders, even when service members are deployed (U.S. DoD and VA, 2014). Implementation of the BHDP throughout the MHS is in different stages, including Navy and Air Force BH clinics (early implementation), traumatic brain injury (TBI) clinics (pilot), BH care integrated in primary care mental health integration (pilot), BH screening in primary care (pilot), and BH evaluations in National Guard Armories (building) (Brown et al., 2015).

The BHDP is an easy-to-use and secure web-based system for collecting behavioral health symptom data directly from patients (Hoge et al., 2015). The system is separate from the electronic health record. It was developed by the Army Medical Command's Behavioral Health Division (Association for Enterprise Information, undated). MEDCOM Policy 14-094 (Department of the Army Headquarters, 2014b) requires the frequency of administration of the PCL to be every 30 days. In contrast, a policy memo from the DoD Working Group on Common Mental Health Metrics suggested that the recommended frequency of administration of the PCL should be "at the initiation of treatment and as clinically indicated during treatment (preferably at each treatment session), but at least once between 60–120 days after intake" (DoD, 2014e). For the PHQ-9, the recommended frequency is "at every clinical encounter where a depressive disorder is the focus of treatment. At a minimum, the PHQ-9 should be administered upon treatment initiation and at least once between 60–120 days after intake" (DoD, 2014e). The questionnaire responses are scored immediately and are available on a provider portal section of BHDP that providers can access from their own computers. Scores and graphing are displayed with color coding to indicate current patient risk and any meaningful changes in risk (Association for Enterprise Information, undated).

Processing Symptom Questionnaire Data

Files of symptom questionnaire data were created by the Behavioral Health Division, Office of the Surgeon General of the Army, and processed by DMDC before they were delivered to RAND. The data in the BHDP files were restricted to Army personnel only and included data for 2013–2015. BHDP includes several patient-reported items available for providers to select for patient completion, including several symptom questionnaires (e.g., PCL, PHQ-9, GAD-7), along with other instruments such as Behavior and Symptom Identification Scale (BASIS-24) and Alcohol Use Disorders Identification Test (AUDIT). Our analyses focused on PTSD and depression symptom scores from the PCL and the PHQ-9. The PCL-Civilian is a 17-item PTSD symptom questionnaire with each item completed by the patient on a 1-to-5 scale ranging from

1 (Not at all) to 5 (Extremely), yielding a total PCL score that can range from 17 to 85. The PHQ-9 is a 9-item depression symptom questionnaire with the patient selecting a response on a 0-to-3 scale to indicate how frequently the symptom occurred during the past two weeks, ranging from 0 (not at all) to 3 (nearly every day), yielding a total score that can range from 0 to 27. We computed a total symptom score for each questionnaire. Each PCL or PHQ-9 score and the date each questionnaire was completed were linked to the administrative data records of soldiers in the PTSD and depression cohorts using their scrambled Social Security number. Some soldiers completed multiple questionnaires during treatment and, therefore, had multiple symptom scores. Other soldiers did not have any symptom scores. The symptom questionnaire data were used in two ways: (1) to calculate scores for six quality measures (Table 2.4), and (2) for multivariate regression analyses described below. For the **calculation of quality measure results**, only PCLs and PHQ-9s with complete data (no missing values) were used. For the **multivariate regression analyses**, if one or two items from the PCL or PHQ-9 were missing, we assigned a score by filling the missing items with the mean of the remaining nonmissing items from the same patient's questionnaire (<1 percent of the PCL scores, and of the PHQ-9 scores). This person-mean imputation approach with two or fewer items missing is more appropriate than removing incomplete questionnaires because of the high internal consistency for both these measures (Graham, 2009). If more than two items were missing, we assigned a missing value to the symptom score (<1 percent of the PCL scores and the PHQ-9 scores).

Symptom Questionnaire Data Quality Measures

We developed or adapted technical specifications for a total of six quality measures that incorporated information from symptom questionnaires (three each for PTSD and for depression); these six measures are listed in Table 2.4. Within the set of symptom questionnaire measures, one measure provides information about the percentage of patients who complete symptom questionnaires on the recommended schedule (T1),

Table 2.4
PTSD and Depression Quality Measures Using Symptom Questionnaire Data

Measure No.	PTSD	Depression
T1	Percentage of PTSD patients with symptom assessment with PCL during 4-month measurement period	Percentage of depression patients with symptom assessment with PHQ-9 during 4-month measurement period[a]
T10	Percentage of PTSD patients (PCL score > 43) with response to treatment (5-point reduction in PCL score) at 6 months	Percentage of depression patients (PHQ-9 score > 9) with response to treatment (50% reduction in PHQ-9 score) at 6 months[a]
T12	Percentage of PTSD patients (PCL score > 43) in PTSD-symptom remission (PCL score < 28) at 6 months	Percentage of depression patients (PHQ-9 score > 9) in depression-symptom remission (PHQ-9 score < 5) at 6 months[a]

[a]NQF-endorsed measure.

and the other two measures are based on the change between baseline and six months in scores using symptom questionnaire data. These changes are classified as response (T10) and remission (T12). PTSD-T10 and T12 are new quality measures, and there are arguments for various PCL score cut points to define the denominators. We chose a score (44) for a broader application of the measure (primary care as well as behavioral health) but still with good specificity and sensitivity (Blanchard et al., 1996). The complete technical specifications for the symptom questionnaire measures are provided in Appendixes A and B for PTSD and depression, respectively.[12] The symptom questionnaire sample used for the quality measures in Table 2.4 was limited to those with direct care only to ensure that measure scores were not lowered due to receipt of care in a purchased care setting that would not be captured in our data sources. Also, because the use of the BHDP was limited to Army behavioral health care at the time of data collection, the symptom questionnaire data used for these measures represent the same subset of patients.

Strengths and Limitations of Symptom Questionnaire Data

The symptom questionnaire data collected through the BHDP offer a way to track clinical outcomes of treatment for PH conditions provided by providers at MTFs. Although separate from the medical record, the BHDP system offers an efficient method of patients completing the questionnaires online and providing feedback to providers immediately for use during patient encounters minutes later. Symptom data are captured in structured fields, making the data easily accessible, when compared with entering this information in an unstructured way in a medical record note. This system collects and analyzes data that allow providers to monitor the progress of individual patients and the MHS to follow cohorts of service members with PH diagnoses over time.

Despite the innovative design and operation of the BHDP system, the data collected by the system have limitations that must be considered in evaluating for what purposes they can be used. First, BHDP is not directly linked to AHLTA, and the provider must therefore either enter the diagnosis for the system to know which symptom questionnaire administration frequency to update or, alternatively, must change the questionnaire frequency directly. If neither of these actions occurs, the patient will be asked to complete a basic screening questionnaire every 60 to 90 days, which may trigger the full symptom questionnaire. Patients do not determine the timing of completion and cannot initiate the process of completion. The provider must also manually enter the symptom score into AHLTA to incorporate it into the documentation of the patient's history of care. BHDP does contain a note template that allows

---

[12]   For each measure in the study, the technical specifications include the following elements: measure title, measure statement, numerator, denominator, measure type, care setting, numerator specifications, denominator specifications, measure source, the rationale for including the measure, and the feasibility of measuring performance from existing data. These are provided in Appendixes A and B for PTSD and depression, respectively.

for easy transfer of symptom questionnaire data into AHLTA. During the time period examined, BHDP was still being adopted with increasing usage, but the inconsistency of use across the enterprise during the implementation period meant that some patients did not have any symptom questionnaire data. In addition, at the time of this study, symptom questionnaires were completed within BHDP only by patients seen in behavioral health specialty care at an MTF, and symptom questionnaires were typically not completed by patients seen in primary care for psychological health conditions within the MTFs or by patients with visits for psychological health conditions with primary care or mental health specialty providers outside of MTFs (i.e., purchased care). The analysis of observational data sources such as the symptom questionnaire data comes with other limitations. An equitable comparison of symptom scores across groups should be adjusted for differences in severity across those groups, so one group does not appear to have worse outcomes simply because one group's patients have greater preexisting severity. Standard risk adjustment approaches such as covariate adjustment in regression are limited to adjusting for known patient characteristics, such as demographics and initial symptom scores, but unobserved or unrecorded differences are not accounted for by standard risk adjustment. Finally, as Army was the developer of BHDP and other service branches were asked to adopt BHDP in 2013, our analyses for this report are limited to Army personnel only. While some data were available for other service branches, the number of questionnaires was not adequate for analysis. When considered together, these factors mean that the symptom score data represent only a subset of the service members with PTSD or depression, which may not be representative of all service members with PTSD or depression. Furthermore, symptom scores of subgroups of service members (e.g., those with initial and six-month follow-up scores within the observation period) may not be representative of all service members with PTSD or depression, or of all service members with a symptom score. For example, of those with an initial PCL score, 32.6 percent had a PCL score five to seven months later. Similarly, of those with an initial PHQ-9 score, 27.6 percent had a PHQ-9 score five to seven months later. Therefore, conclusions based on symptom questionnaire data collected through the BHDP should be interpreted cautiously and may not apply to the group as a whole.

Analyses

As described in the sections above, we analyzed data from three sources: administrative data, medical record data, and symptom questionnaire data. In this section, we describe how the three sources were used in the analyses presented in the report.

Description of Service Member Characteristics Based on Administrative Data

Using administrative data, we describe service members in the PTSD and depression cohorts in terms of demographic characteristics (gender, age, race/ethnicity, and marital status), service characteristics (branch of service, pay grade, years of service, deployment history, and geographic region), and health care utilization characteristics (treatment setting, characteristics of the care delivered, and types of treatment provided). We also describe the care received by the system of care used (i.e., direct or purchased care), the primary condition being treated (cohort condition, other PH condition, or non-PH condition), and the prevalence of co-occurring conditions. For these analyses, we present descriptive statistics, including percentages, means, medians, standard deviations, and ranges with minimums and maximums.

Quality Measure Scores

To describe the quality of care for PTSD and depression delivered by the MHS, we computed measure scores for each quality measure using administrative data, medical record data, or symptom questionnaire data. The numerator (i.e., the process of the care recommended in the measure) and denominator (i.e., individuals eligible for the recommended care) of each quality measure were calculated from the appropriate data source during the identified 12-month observation period for each service member. Each measure score is a percentage or mean equal to the value resulting from the measure numerator being divided by the measure denominator. Note that while the period of time during which care was observed was January 1, 2013 through June 30, 2014, data from 2012 were used for selected measures to determine denominator eligibility (e.g., check for a "clean period" prior to the start of a new treatment episode). Detailed technical specifications for each quality measure are available in Appendixes A and B for PTSD and depression, respectively. In the discussion of the results in Chapters Four and Five, we present related quality measure scores from other health care systems and from published literature, when available, to provide a context for the results presented in this study. The processing and use of the symptom questionnaire data for analysis of quality measure scores differed from the processing and use in the multivariate regression analyses (described below). Table 2.5 compares the use of these data for these two analyses, quality measures versus multivariate regression analyses (Analyses of Symptom Questionnaire Data described later).

Variations in Quality Measure Scores Using Administrative Data

To assess equity of care provided by the MHS, we analyzed quality measure scores based on administrative data by sociodemographic and service characteristics wherever quality measure denominator sizes permitted[13]. The Institute of Medicine con-

---

[13] Due to the relatively low numbers of service members eligible for T10 and T12, variations in performance by sociodemographic and service characteristics were not examined. Thus, these two measure scores are estimated

Table 2.5
Comparison of Quality Measure Analyses and Multivariate Regression Analyses Using Symptom Questionnaire Data

Data Characteristics	Quality Measure Analyses	Multivariate Regression Analyses
Source of data	BHDP	BHDP
Branch of service	Army	Army
Use of care during analysis period	Direct care only	Direct and/or purchased care
Type of visits	Behavioral health	Behavioral health
Dates of care included	January 2013–June 2014	January 2013–June 2014
Missing data items in PCL or PHQ-9	Scores with any missing items were excluded	**One or two items missing:** Missing item values imputed **More than two items missing:** Missing value assigned to symptom score
Requirements for eligibility	**Measure T1:** Required one condition-related encounter in the four–month measurement period **Measures T10/T12:** Required one condition-related encounter and a symptom score above a measure-defined threshold in the first five months of the 12-month measurement period	Required two symptom scores (initial and five to seven months later)
Adjustment for confounders	No	Yes
Statistical testing conducted	No	Yes
Relationship with process quality measures evaluated	No	Yes

siders equity to be one of the domains of health care quality (Institute of Medicine, 2001). Care that is equitable does not vary in quality by patient characteristics, such as gender, racial/ethnic background, and geographic location. Therefore, for quality measures based on administrative data, we examined differences in scores by service branch (Army, Air Force, Marine Corps, Navy) and TRICARE region (North, South, West, Overseas). Scores were also computed for the following service member subgroups: age,

for the study population overall. If denominators were sufficiently large to examine variations, then risk adjustment could be considered to compare measure scores while controlling for differences across service member characteristic categories. However, the specifications for risk adjustment developed by Minnesota Community Measurement for the NQF-endorsed Measure No. 0711 (National Quality Forum, 2015a) would need to be modified for the service member population; for example, the existing risk adjustment specifications include adjustment for patient distance from clinic and insurance type.

race/ethnicity, gender, pay grade, and history of deployment at time of cohort entry. Age was defined as of the time of cohort entry based on age categories (18–24 years, 25–34 years, 35–44 years, and 45–64 years). Service members 65 years and older were not included in these analyses due to small numbers still on active duty. Race/ethnicity was obtained from the Defense Manpower Data Center (DMDC) database. While we present more detailed information in describing the cohorts, we created four collapsed race/ethnicity categories to allow sufficient numbers to analyze variations: white, non-Hispanic; black, non-Hispanic; Hispanic (including white/Hispanic; black/Hispanic; American Indian or Alaskan native/Hispanic; Asian or Pacific Islander/Hispanic; and race unknown/Hispanic), and Other/Unknown (including American Indian/Alaskan Native; Asian or Pacific Islander; Multiracial; and Unknown). We analyzed measure scores for female and male service members, and four subgroups classified by pay grade: E1–E4; E5–E9, O1–O3, and O4–O6. Service members in C1, O7–O8, and warrant categories of pay grade were not included in these analyses due to small numbers. Using information about deployment from the DMDC database (Contingency Tracking System–Deployments), we compared measure scores between those with no deployments at the time of cohort entry and those with one or more deployments. We examined variation in measure scores by these characteristics for all measures.

Most quality measures are specified so that each individual in the denominator is assigned either 0 or 1 for not having or having the care specified in the numerator, respectively. To allow for the possibility of a small number of individuals being eligible for these measures for some subgroups, we performed a Fisher's exact test to test for statistically significant differences between measure scores in these subgroups. We report multiplicity-adjusted P-values to account for the fact we are conducting a large number of statistical tests. If we were to assume the commonly used P-value cutoff of 0.05 to identify statistically significant results, we would expect 5 percent of all tests to be statistically significant by chance alone, even in the absence of true differences. The adjusted P-values reported in Appendix D control the false discovery rate (the proportion of statistically significant findings that are false positives) (Benjamini and Hochberg, 1995) to be 5 percent.

Analyses of Symptom Questionnaire Data

We restricted all analyses of symptom questionnaire data to Army personnel due to the limited use of the BHDP system by behavioral health clinics in the other service branches in 2013–2014. We conducted analyses to describe the relationship between the number of completed symptom questionnaires and the number of mental health specialty visits for the entire 12-month observation period. We also calculated the symptom questionnaire completion rate on a monthly basis as the number of symptom questionnaires completed per 100 mental health specialty visits.[14] For Army personnel in the PTSD or depression cohorts, we ran chi-squared and t-tests to examine whether there were significant differences in member and service characteristics between two subgroups defined by completing two or more symptom questionnaires versus completing one or none. As noted earlier and in Table 2.5, the processing and use of these data for these analyses differed from the methods using these data for calculation of quality measure scores.

We conducted two sets of analyses. First, we examined whether there were significant changes in symptom scores (PCL or PHQ-9) six months after the initial score by fitting repeated measures multivariable linear regression models to the initial and six-month symptom scores. The following variables were covariates in the model: age (18–24, 25–34, 35–44, 45 and older), male (0,1), race/ethnicity (white, non-Hispanic; black, non-Hispanic; Hispanic; other), pay grade (E1–E4, E5–E9, O1–O3, O4–O8),[15] region (north, south, west, overseas), Charlson Comorbidity Index, number of years of service, and an indicator of measurement time of the symptom score (0 = initial, 1 = six months). Standard error estimates were adjusted to account for the nonindependence of repeated observations for each person. The statistical significance of the change in symptoms over time was assessed by examining the regression coefficient estimate of the measurement time indicator. To adjust for differences on the observed covariates for those with versus without six-month follow-up data, the regression analyses were weighted to represent everyone receiving direct behavioral mental health specialty care. Weights were estimated as the reciprocal of the predicted probability of having six-month follow-up data (Kim and Kim, 2007). The predicted probabilities were estimated using logistic regression of an indicator of having symptom data observed at six months as the dependent variable and the independent variables of age (18–24, 25–34, 35–44, 45 and older), male (0,1), race/ethnicity (white, non-Hispanic; black, non-Hispanic; Hispanic; other), pay grade (E1–E4, E5–E9, O1–O3, O4–O8), region (north south, west, overseas), Charlson Comorbidity Index, and number of years of service. Second, we evaluated whether receipt of evidence-based care is associated with a change in symptom scores (PCL or PHQ-9) six months after the initial score using multivariable regression models. The linear regression model was set up with the symptom score at six months as the dependent variable, and the following variables as covariates in the model: the initial symptom score (continuous) and the covariates listed above. The statistical significance of the association between the quality measure

---

[14] Mental health specialty visits were restricted to direct care and identified on the basis of the Medical Expense & Performance Reporting System (MEPRS3) variable in the Comprehensive Ambulatory Professional Encounter (CAPER) file. The following categories were excluded from the count of mental health specialty visits: group therapy, family therapy, teleconference, and any visits with an "Appointment Status" not equal to kept, walk-in, or sick call.

[15] Due to few persons being in O7–O8, the O7–O8 categories were combined with the O4–O6 categories for the multivariate analyses.

and adjusted symptoms change score was assessed by examining the regression coefficient estimate of the quality measure. Analyses were weighted as above to represent the population of those who received mental health specialty care who were eligible for at least one of the quality measures.

CHAPTER THREE

Characteristics of Service Members in PTSD and Depression Cohorts, and Their Care Settings and Treatments

In this chapter, we describe the demographic and service characteristics of service members in the PTSD and depression cohorts using administrative data. We then detail the settings in which these service members received their health care, as well as the types of care received. We describe what care was provided to each individual in the cohorts during an observation period of 12 months. For each service member included in the cohort, the 12-month observation period occurred during January 2013 through June 2014 and was initiated by receiving an outpatient visit or inpatient stay with a cohort diagnosis (i.e., PTSD or depression).

The findings presented in this chapter are not intended to be a direct comparison between service members with PTSD and those with depression, in part because of the substantial amount of overlap between the two cohorts (i.e., 6,322 service members were in both cohorts, representing 43.1 percent of the PTSD cohort and 20.7 percent of the depression cohort). We do not report results for the subgroup of service members included in both cohorts separately. However, Table 3.3 highlights the prevalence of co-occurring conditions, and we briefly note the percentage of each cohort that has the other cohort diagnosis at some point during the observation period.

We reported similar analyses in a prior report for an earlier observation period (i.e., care delivered from January 2012 through June 2013) (Hepner et al., 2016). The reader will note that the descriptive results presented here are largely similar to those presented in the prior report, suggesting that the characteristics of service members with PTSD or depression and the nature of the care they received did not change in the more recent period (i.e., care delivered from January 2013 through June 2014). Further, it is important to note that many service members appear in both the 2012–2013 and 2013–2014 cohorts. Over a quarter of service members in the 2013–2014 PTSD cohort (28 percent) were also in the 2012–2013 PTSD cohort, and one-fourth of those in the 2013–2014 depression cohort (26 percent) were also in the 2012–2013 depression cohort. Despite similar results and some overlap in the population with the prior report, we detail the complete set of descriptive findings to fully characterize the service members of this study and the care they received in a more recent time period.

Demographic Characteristics of the PTSD and Depression Cohorts

Table 3.1 shows the majority of service members in the PTSD cohort were white, non-Hispanic males, with nearly half the cohort between 25 and 34 years of age. Individuals in this cohort were geographically well distributed throughout the TRICARE regions. About a third of participants resided in TRICARE South, another third were located in TRICARE West. Furthermore, approximately one-fifth were based in TRI-CARE North, and the remainder were overseas or in an unknown location. Only a very small subgroup (2 percent) was living in geographic areas considered remote according to TRICARE's definition. The depression cohort exhibited a similar pattern of characteristics as the PTSD cohort (Table 3.1). However, a larger percentage of the depression cohort was female, younger, and never married.

Table 3.1
Demographic Characteristics of PTSD and Depression Cohorts, 2013–2014

Demographic Characteristic	PTSD Cohort % (n) (n = 14,654)	Depression Cohort % (n) (n = 30,496)
Gender		
Female	19.2 (2,819)	33.6 (10,239)
Male	80.8 (11,835)	66.4 (20,257)
Age at diagnosis		
18–24	14.8 (2,175)	23.2 (7,069)
25–34	45.3 (6,644)	44.0 (13,424)
35–44	33.8 (4,954)	27.6 (8,428)
45–64	6.0 (881)	5.2 (1,575)
Race/ethnicity		
American Indian/Alaskan Native	1.5 (213)	1.4 (436)
Asian/Pacific Islander	4.8 (700)	4.4 (1,327)
Black, non-Hispanic	20.0 (2,927)	19.4 (5,929)
White, non-Hispanic	58.6 (8,581)	60.3 (18,385)
Hispanic	13.1 (1,924)	11.7 (3,579)
Multiracial/multiethnic	0.6 (86)	0.6 (190)
Unknown	1.5 (223)	2.1 (650)

Table 3.1—Continued

Demographic Characteristic	PTSD Cohort % (n) (n = 14,654)	Depression Cohort % (n) (n = 30,496)
Marital status		
Married	75.7 (11,099)	65.7 (20,037)
Never married	13.6 (1,988)	23.1 (7,039)
Divorced, separated, widowed	10.7 (1,567)	11.2 (3,418)
Unknown	0 (0)	(NR)
Region		
TRICARE North	21.1 (3,096)	24.9 (7,604)
TRICARE South	34.3 (5,019)	29.7 (9,044)
TRICARE West	32.1 (4,705)	32.6 (9,931)
TRICARE Overseas	10.4 (1,518)	11.1 (3,398)
Unknown	2.2 (316)	1.7 (519)
Remote/rural		
Not remote	97.9 (14,350)	97.7 (29,792)
Remote[a]	2.1 (304)	2.3 (704)

NOTE: PTSD and depression cohorts are not mutually exclusive. NR = not reported (cells with fewer than five).

[a] Based on eligibility flag for TRICARE Prime Remote.

Military Service Characteristics of the PTSD and Depression Cohorts

Table 3.2 shows the military service characteristics of members of both the PTSD and depression cohorts. Service members in the Army constituted 69 percent of the PTSD cohort, while Air Force, Marine Corps, and Navy represented 12, 11, and 8 percent of the cohort, respectively. Given that in 2013, 39 percent of all active-duty service members were Army, with 24 percent Air Force, 23 percent Navy, and 14 percent Marines (DoD, 2014d), it is clear that Army is overrepresented among those diagnosed with PTSD. Enlisted service members represented 89 percent of the PTSD cohort, and 51 percent of the PTSD cohort had ten or fewer years of service at the time of cohort entry. About 90 percent of the PTSD cohort had been deployed at least once, and the average service member had 20 cumulative months of deployment at the time of cohort entry.

Table 3.2
Service Characteristics of the PTSD and Depression Cohorts, 2013–2014

Service Characteristic	PTSD Cohort % (n) (n = 14, 654)	Depression Cohort % (n) (n = 30, 496)
Service branch		
Army	68.5 (10,045)	55.7 (16,980)
Air Force	11.5 (1,692)	19.1 (5,833)
Marine Corps	10.5 (1,543)	8.5 (2,601)
Navy	8.5 (1,245)	14.0 (4,280)
Coast Guard	0.9 (129)	2.6 (802)
Rank		
C1, E1–E4	25.1 (3,675)	35.3 (10,776)
E5–E9	64.3 (9,417)	52.0 (15,857)
O1–O3	4.1 (601)	5.7 (1,725)
O4–O8	4.5 (661)	5.5 (1,686)
Warrant	2.0 (300)	1.5 (452)
Years of service		
0–3	10.3 (1,510)	21.4 (6,535)
4–6	17.2 (2,514)	19.1 (5,817)
7–10	23.5 (3,439)	19.5 (5,950)
11–15	20.9 (3,060)	17.5 (5,331)
16–20	19.9 (2,909)	16.4 (5,003)
More than 20	8.3 (1,218)	6.1 (1,851)
Unknown	NR	NR
Deployment experience[a]		
Ever deployed	89.9 (13,176)	68.0 (20,751)
Number of deployments at time of cohort entry[a]		
None	10.1 (1,478)	32.0 (9,745)
1–3	75.0 (10,992)	60.0 (18,294)
4–6	14.2 (2,074)	7.7 (2,344)
7 or more	0.8 (110)	0.4 (113)

Table 3.2—Continued

Service Characteristic	PTSD Cohort % (n) (n = 14, 654)	Depression Cohort % (n) (n = 30, 496)
Months deployed at time of cohort entry[a]		
Mean (min, max)	20.3 (0.03, 91.9)	16.6 (0.03, 84.1)
Median	18.5	12.8
Mode	11.9	11.7

NOTE: PTSD and depression cohorts are not mutually exclusive. NR = not reported (cells with fewer than five).

[a] Based on data from September 2001 through March 2015.

While active service members in the Army represented 56 percent of the depression cohort, individuals in the Air Force, Marine Corps, and Navy contributed 19, 9, and 14 percent, respectively, to this cohort. Given the 2013 breakdown by service for all active-duty service members—39 percent Army, 24 percent Air Force, 23 percent Navy, and 14 percent Marines (DoD, 2014d)—Army is slightly overrepresented among those with a depression diagnosis. Nearly 90 percent of service members in the depression cohort were enlisted. Approximately one-fifth of the depression cohort had three or fewer years of service. More than two-thirds of individuals in the depression cohort had been deployed at least once at the time of cohort entry, with a cumulative average of 17 months.

Sources of Care for PTSD and Depression

We investigated which sources of care service members in the PTSD and depression cohorts used. First, we describe the percentage of patients who received treatment for mental health conditions as direct care, purchased care, or both. Each record in the patient encounter files contains all diagnoses for that clinic visit or hospitalization.

The results in Figures 3.1 and 3.2 represent all outpatient and inpatient encounters for which the cohort diagnosis (PTSD or depression) was recorded, irrespective of its position (i.e., primary or secondary). Figure 3.1 depicts how members of the PTSD cohort are broken down by the source (i.e., direct or purchased care) of their outpatient and inpatient care with a PTSD diagnosis. About 22 percent of the PTSD cohort received both direct and purchased care, with nearly 12 percent receiving more than 50 percent direct care, and approximately 10 percent receiving less than or equal to 50 percent direct care.

Figure 3.2 shows the breakdown of members of the depression cohort by source of their outpatient and inpatient encounters with a depression diagnosis. More than

Figure 3.1
Service Members in the PTSD Cohort, by Source of Care for Inpatient and Outpatient Encounters with PTSD Diagnoses, 2013–2014

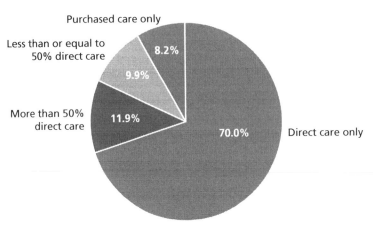

RAND RR1542-3.1

Figure 3.2
Service Members in the Depression Cohort, by Source of Care for Inpatient and Outpatient Encounters with Depression Diagnoses, 2013–2014

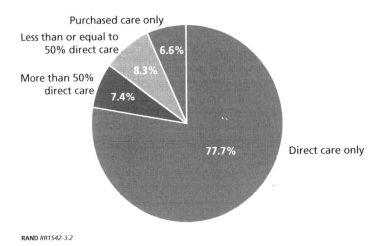

RAND RR1542-3.2

three-quarters of service members in the depression cohort received care for their depression only at MTFs ("direct care only" in Figure 3.2). Nearly 7 percent of the cohort received solely purchased care for this diagnosis. Nearly 16 percent of individuals in this cohort received care from both direct care and purchased care—7.4 percent of the cohort received more than 50 percent direct care, and 8.3 percent received less than or equal to 50 percent direct care.

Next we combined direct and purchased care to investigate the primary diagnoses coded during each patient encounter for members of the PTSD and depression cohorts. Up to 20 diagnoses can be assigned to an encounter, depending on the type of encounter, and the primary diagnosis may or may not truly represent the key issue addressed during the encounter. To address these issues, we defined three distinct classifications for primary diagnoses:

- *Primary diagnosis—PTSD/depression*: The primary diagnosis was the condition by which the service member entered the cohort (PTSD if in the PTSD cohort, depression if in the depression cohort)
- *Primary diagnosis—other PH*: The primary diagnosis was a PH condition other than the condition for which the service member was included in the cohort[1]
- *Primary diagnosis—non-PH*: The primary diagnosis was a condition not included in the two categories listed above (i.e., general medical or surgical conditions or preventive care).

As Figure 3.3 illustrates, the majority of encounters for service members in the PTSD cohort were for a non-psychological health condition primary diagnosis (i.e. medical care).[2] However, 43 percent of all encounters for the PTSD cohort involved

Figure 3.3
Primary Diagnoses for All Patient Encounters for the PTSD Cohort, 2013–2014

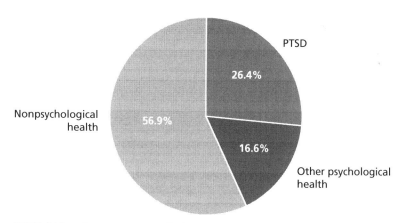

NOTE: "All patient encounters" includes direct and purchased care.
RAND RR1542-3.3

---

[1] ICD-9-CM codes that define "other psychological health condition" are 290.xx–319.xx, excluding the codes that define the PTSD and depression cohorts listed in Appendixes A and B, respectively, available online: http://www.rand.org/pubs/research_reports/RR1542.html.

[2] Our analysis did not focus on what medical conditions were co-occurring with the cohort condition. In the next section, we describe co-occurring mental health conditions, and in that discussion, we mention only one non–mental health condition (traumatic brain injury).

a PTSD or another psychological health diagnosis, with 26 percent of all encounters including a primary diagnosis for PTSD. The primary diagnoses for patient encounters in the depression cohort followed a similar pattern in that the majority of primary diagnoses for this cohort were for non-psychological health conditions (Figure 3.4). However, while almost 41 percent of all encounters were for depression or another psychological health condition, a smaller percentage (16 percent) had a primary diagnosis of depression. There are several possible reasons for the lower percentage with a primary diagnosis of depression in the depression cohort than PTSD in the PTSD cohort. Perhaps this reflects a higher likelihood of a provider perceiving depression as secondary to a general medical condition (thus resulting in a reduced probability of coding depression as the primary diagnosis). This difference may also be partially attributable to having a broader number of diagnosis codes beyond MDD included in the depression definition, with the MDD code having a higher likelihood of being assigned as a primary diagnosis than the other depression diagnosis codes included in the depression cohort definition. Furthermore, given the overlap between the PTSD and depression cohorts, it may also be that individuals in the depression cohort with comorbid PTSD received a primary PTSD diagnosis, while depression was relegated to the secondary position.

Figure 3.4
Primary Diagnoses for All Patient Encounters for the Depression Cohort, 2013–2014

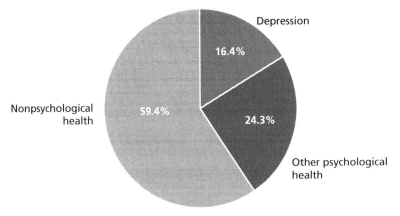

NOTE: "All patient encounters" includes direct and purchased care.
RAND RR1542-3.3

Comorbid Psychological Health Conditions

We examined the proportion of service members in each cohort who received services for other selected psychological health conditions[3] during the observation period (i.e., the 12 months following entry into the cohort). The two most common comorbid conditions within the PTSD cohort were sleep disorders/symptoms (60 percent) and depression (55 percent). The number of service members in the PTSD cohort with comorbid depression (n = 7,991) represents comorbidity over the entire 12-month observation period. As such, this number is higher than the number in the PTSD cohort who also entered the depression cohort (n = 6,322), which was limited to the six-month cohort entry window. Anxiety and adjustment disorders were also common among these service members and were diagnosed in 47 and 35 percent of the PTSD cohort, respectively. While our primary focus for this section concerns psychological health disorders, we also examined the proportion of patients within the PTSD cohort with a diagnosis of TBI.[4] We identified 2,104 members of the cohort (14.4 percent) who received a TBI diagnosis (not shown).

The percentages with psychological health comorbidity within the depression cohort were largely similar to those of the PTSD cohort. Large percentages of the depression cohort received a sleep disorders/symptoms diagnosis (46 percent), anxiety disorders diagnosis (43 percent), adjustment disorders diagnosis (39 percent), and 27 percent of this cohort (n = 8,126) received a comorbid PTSD diagnosis during the observation window. Again, this number is higher than the number also in the PTSD cohort (n = 6,322) for the aforementioned reasons. Note that a substantially smaller portion of the depression cohort received a sleep disorder/symptoms diagnosis (46 percent) when compared with that of the PTSD cohort (60 percent). Although not shown in Table 3.3, 6.5 percent of the depression cohort (n = 1,983) received a TBI diagnosis.

---

[3]   ICD-9-CM codes (primary or secondary) used to define comorbid PH conditions were the following: acute stress disorders: 308.x; adjustment disorders: 309.xx (excludes 309.1, 309.21, 309.22, 309.23, 309.81); alcohol abuse/dependence: 305.0x, 303.xx; anxiety disorders: 300.00–300.10, 300.2x, 300.3, 300.5, 300.89, 300.9; attention deficit disorder: 314.xx; bipolar disorder: 296.0x, 296.1x, 296.4x, 296.5x, 296.6x, 296.7xx, 296.8x (excludes 296.90); depression: 296.2x, 296.3x, 293.83, 296.90, 296.99, 298.0, 300.4, 309.1, 311; drug abuse/dependence: 304.xx, 305.2x–305.9x; personality disorders: 301.xx; posttraumatic stress disorder (PTSD): 309.81; sleep disorders/symptoms: 327.xx, 347.xx, 307.4x, 780.5x.

[4]   ICD-9-CM codes (primary or secondary) used to define TBI were the following: 800.xx, 801.xx, 803.xx, 804.xx, 850.xx, 851.xx, 852.0x–852.5x, 853.0x, 853.1x, 854.0x, 854.1x, 310.2, 950.1–950.3, 959.01, V80.01, V15.52.

Table 3.3
Comorbid Psychological Health Conditions in the PTSD and Depression Cohorts, 2013–2014

Diagnosis	PTSD Cohort % (n) (n = 14,654)	Depression Cohort % (n) (n = 30,496)
Acute stress disorder	2.1 (312)	2.1 (630)
Adjustment disorders	34.5 (5,060)	39.4 (12,003)
Alcohol abuse/dependence	15.6 (2,290)	13.3 (4,043)
Anxiety disorders	47.3 (6,930)	42.8 (13,040)
Attention deficit disorder	8.2 (1,199)	9.3 (2,824)
Bipolar disorder	3.2 (464)	3.5 (1,077)
Depression	54.5 (7,991)	100 (30,496)
Drug abuse/dependence	5.6 (814)	4.4 (1,351)
Personality disorders	4.5 (653)	5.3 (1,607)
PTSD	100 (14,654)	26.6 (8,126)
Sleep disorders/symptoms	60.2 (8,818)	45.7 (13,928)

NOTES: Includes direct and purchased care. PTSD and depression cohorts are not mutually exclusive.

Treatment Setting, Encounter Characteristics, and Types of Providers Seen by PTSD and Depression Patients

In this section, we describe the settings in which members of the PTSD and depression cohorts received treatment for PTSD or depression. Table 3.4 details the percentage of service members in each cohort who received mental health care, primary care, subspecialty care and/or emergency care in one of these outpatient settings coded with

Table 3.4
Percentage of PTSD and Depression Cohort Patients Who Received Outpatient Care Associated with a PTSD or Depression Diagnosis, by Direct and Purchased Care, 2013–2014

Outpatient Care	PTSD Cohort		Depression Cohort	
	Direct Care[a]	Purchased Care[b]	Direct Care[a]	Purchased Care[b]
Mental Health	76.3	20.7	67.3	12.8
Primary Care	46.7	3.4	48.0	2.9
Subspecialty	12.2	2.5	7.0	2.1
Emergency	2.6	1.2	5.9	2.9

NOTE: PTSD and depression cohorts are not mutually exclusive.

[a] Based on CAPER MEPRS

[b] Based on TED-NI Product Line

the cohort diagnosis. We chose to include visits with a cohort diagnosis listed in the primary or secondary position (instead of restricting to the primary position) because assigning a diagnosis, regardless of position, suggests that the condition may have been treated during the encounter. Given the high percentages with psychological and physical health comorbidities, PTSD and depression are likely to be treated alongside co-occurring conditions. We opted to include visits where the cohort diagnosis was listed as secondary to capture such encounters.

Results are shown separately for direct and purchased care. Individuals may be included in multiple cells of the table (for example, if the same service member received care at a MTF subspecialty clinic and at a community based primary care clinic). Over three-fourths of patients in the PTSD cohort visited mental health clinics at MTFs, and nearly half of the cohort received care from MTF primary care clinics. While one-fifth of PTSD patients were seen in a mental health setting under purchased care, few members of this cohort received PTSD care through purchased care from clinics other than mental health.

More than two-thirds of patients in the depression cohort received care for depression in MTF mental health clinics. Similar to those in the PTSD cohort, almost half of all depression cohort patients were seen at MTF primary care clinics. Fewer patients in the depression cohort used purchased care than direct care in all outpatient settings. These findings suggest that while many patients in both cohorts present to MTF mental health clinics for care, a considerable proportion of patients also receive treatment related to the cohort diagnosis from primary care providers at MTFs.

Characteristics of Inpatient Stays

This section details the characteristics of inpatient stays among PTSD and depression cohort patients who received inpatient care from direct or purchased care. In Table 3.5, we describe the percentage of service members who had an inpatient stay, the number of discharges per 1,000 in each cohort, and the median length of patient stay based on direct and purchased care. One in five patients in the PTSD cohort had at least one inpatient stay for any diagnosis during the observation period, and 15 percent of the PTSD cohort had an inpatient stay specifically related to PTSD. There were 303 inpatient discharges for every 1,000 patients in the cohort, of which 98 per 1,000 had a primary diagnosis of PTSD, 81 per 1,000 had a primary diagnosis of another psychological health condition, and 124 per 1,000 had a primary diagnosis of a non-psychological health condition. We then investigated the length of acute inpatient stays for individuals within each cohort. For PTSD cohort patients with a primary PTSD discharge diagnosis, the median length of hospitalization stay per admission was 25 days. Stays for other psychological health and medical diagnoses were substantially shorter (seven and two days, respectively). Lastly, two-thirds (66 percent) of inpatient stays among those in the PTSD cohort had a cohort diagnosis in one of the discharge diagnosis fields (primary or secondary).

Table 3.5
Characteristics of Acute Inpatient Care in the PTSD and Depression Cohorts, 2013–2014

Care Characteristic	PTSD Cohort	Depression Cohort
Percentage of cohort patients with any inpatient care	21.3	21.9
Acute inpatient discharges per 1,000 patients, total	303	300
Primary diagnosis—PTSD/depression	98	101
Primary diagnosis—other psychological health	81	68
Primary diagnosis—non-psychological health	124	131
Acute inpatient length of stay (median days per admission)		
Primary diagnosis—PTSD/depression	25	7
Primary diagnosis—other psychological health	7	7
Primary diagnosis—non-psychological health	2	2

NOTES: Inpatient care includes direct and purchased care. PTSD and depression cohorts are not mutually exclusive.

Similar to the PTSD cohort, approximately 20 percent of patients in the depression cohort received inpatient care, including direct and purchased care, for any diagnosis during the observation period (Table 3.5). Of the 300 acute inpatient discharges per 1,000 patients, 101 per 1,000 had a primary diagnosis of depression, 68 per 1,000 had a primary diagnosis of another psychological health condition, and 131 per 1,000 had a primary diagnosis of a non-psychological health condition. Approximately 14 percent of the depression cohort had an inpatient stay related to depression. Hospitalizations for members of the depression cohort with a primary discharge diagnosis of depression had a median length of stay of seven days, as did those with another psychological health diagnosis. The median length of stay for depression cohort patients admitted with a primary diagnosis of a non-psychological health condition was substantially shorter, at two days. Nearly 60 percent of all inpatient stays experienced by depression cohort members noted depression as one of the discharge diagnoses.

Characteristics of Outpatient Encounters

This section details the characteristics of outpatient encounters among PTSD and depression cohort patients who received outpatient care across direct and purchased care. In Table 3.6, we show the utilization of outpatient care (direct and purchased care) among the PTSD and depression cohorts. First, we examined all outpatient encounters of patients in each cohort, irrespective of whether the diagnostic code assigned to the visit matched the condition criteria for cohort inclusion (PTSD or depression). Outpatient visits were counted separately based on provider type, regardless of day of service.

Table 3.6
Characteristics of Outpatient Care in the PTSD and Depression Cohorts, 2013–2014

Care Characteristic	PTSD Cohort	Depression Cohort
Percentage of patients with any outpatient encounters (any diagnosis)	100.0	100.0
Outpatient encounters (any diagnosis)		
Mean (per patient)	51.4	40.0
Median (per patient)	40	31
Number of outpatient encounters, median (total encounters)		
Primary diagnosis—PTSD/depression	10	4
Primary diagnosis—other psychological health	6	8
Primary diagnosis—non-psychological health	22	18

NOTES: Outpatient care includes direct and purchased care. PTSD and depression cohorts are not mutually exclusive.

Accordingly, patients could have visits with more than one provider per calendar day.[5] Even though service members could qualify for the cohort with either an inpatient stay or an outpatient visit with a PTSD diagnosis, all PTSD patients had at least one outpatient encounter during the 12-month observation period. Overall, PTSD patients demonstrated a high level of outpatient service utilization, as members of this cohort averaged nearly one encounter per week for any reason (i.e., medical or psychological) during the 12-month observation period. Yet just one-third (33 percent) of all outpatient encounters for members of the PTSD cohort included PTSD as either a primary or secondary diagnosis (not shown).

We then investigated the median number of outpatient visits that occurred during the course of the year by primary diagnosis. Individuals within the PTSD cohort had a median of 10 outpatient encounters with a primary PTSD diagnosis, a median of six outpatient visits with a primary diagnosis related to another psychological health conditions, and a median of 22 outpatient visits with a non–psychological health primary care diagnosis.

Now, we focus on outpatient visits based on direct and purchased care for members of the depression cohort (Table 3.6). Patients in this cohort had an average of 40 outpatient visits for any diagnosis during the 12-month observation period. Nearly one-fourth (23 percent) of all outpatient visits for the depression cohort included depression as a diagnosis (either the primary or secondary; not shown). The number of outpatient encounters among the depression cohort varied by primary diagnosis. Among the depression cohort, the median number of encounters with a primary non-

---

[5]   See the appendix in the Phase I report (Hepner et al., 2016) for the detailed methods related to counting encounters by provider type.

psychological health diagnosis (18) was substantially higher than the median number of encounters coded with a primary diagnosis of depression or other psychological health conditions (four and eight encounters, respectively).

Types of Providers Seen by Members of the PTSD and Depression Cohorts

In Figures 3.5 and 3.6, we characterize the type of providers who delivered care to members of the PTSD and depression cohorts for **outpatient encounters that have the cohort diagnosis in either a primary or secondary position in direct or purchased care, regardless of outpatient setting.** Patients in both the depression and PTSD cohorts saw a wide variety of providers. In both cohorts, over half of patients received care from primary care providers. Social workers, psychiatrists, and clinical psychologists each provided care for slightly less than half of the PTSD cohort. In contrast, each of these mental health provider groups saw between 33 and 40 percent of the depression cohort. Other medical providers delivered care to 18 percent and 15 percent of patients in the PTSD and depression cohorts, respectively, and other mental health providers (excluding the aforementioned social workers, clinical psychologists, and psychiatrists) served 16 percent of the PTSD cohort, and 12 percent of the depression cohort. The median number of unique providers seen by cohort patients during the observation year at encounters with a cohort diagnosis (coded in any position) was three for PTSD and two for depression. Only 4 percent of all direct care cohort-related visits were provided by a behavioral health provider (i.e., psychiatrist, clinical

Figure 3.5
Percentage of Patients in the PTSD Cohort Who Received Outpatient Care Associated with a PTSD Diagnosis, by Provider Type, 2013–2014

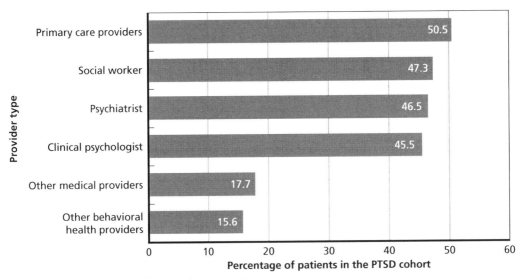

NOTE: Includes providers in direct and purchased care.

RAND RR1542-3.5

Figure 3.6
Percentage of Patients in the Depression Cohort Who Received Outpatient Care Associated with a Depression Diagnosis, by Provider Type, 2013–2014

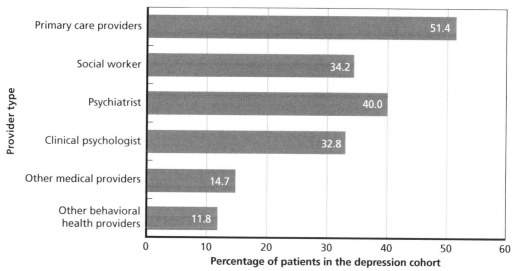

NOTE: Includes providers in direct and purchased care.
RAND *RR1542-3.6*

psychologist/psychoanalyst, clinical social worker, or psychiatric nurse practitioner) in a primary care setting. When considering all outpatient encounters (for any reason), the median number of unique providers was 14 for PTSD and 12 for depression. Given that, it is critical for researchers to thoroughly examine these treatment utilization patterns in future analyses to better inform care coordination and patient management efforts.

Behavioral Assessment Services Delivered to Service Members in the PTSD and Depression Cohorts

Members of the PTSD and depression cohorts received numerous types of assessments (for any diagnosis) (Table 3.7). While three-quarters of the PTSD cohort received psychiatric diagnostic evaluation or psychological testing (with an average of nearly four sessions per patient), nearly 70 percent of the depression cohort received these assessments and averaged three sessions per patient. A much smaller portion of the PTSD cohort (11 percent) and the depression cohort (6 percent) received neuropsychological testing. Health and behavior assessments were performed on 12 percent of the PTSD cohort and 9 percent of the depression cohort, while telephone assessment and management (non–physician qualified) was completed with 5 percent and 3 percent of the PTSD and depression cohorts, respectively.

Table 3.7
Percentage of Patients in PTSD and Depression Cohorts Receiving Assessments, 2013–2014

Assessment	PTSD Cohort		Depression Cohort	
	Percentage of Patients Who Received Service	Mean Number of Sessions	Percentage of Patients Who Received Service	Mean Number of Sessions
Psychiatric diagnostic evaluation/ psychological testing	75.4	3.5	69.8	3.1
Neuropsychological testing	10.7	1.6	5.7	1.5
Health and behavior assessment	12.0	2.4	8.6	2.0
Telephone assessment and management: non–physician qualified	4.5	1.8	3.1	1.8

NOTES: Includes direct and purchased care. PTSD and depression cohorts are not mutually exclusive.

Behavioral Interventions Delivered to Service Members in the PTSD and Depression Cohorts

We now characterize selected treatments administered to members of the PTSD and depression cohorts. First, we report the percentage of patients within each cohort who received any psychotherapy (associated with any diagnosis), and for those recipients, present the average number of sessions attended. As shown in Table 3.8, a high percentage of both the PTSD and depression cohorts completed at least one visit that included psychotherapy—91 percent and 83 percent, respectively. Individual psychotherapy was the most commonly used treatment modality in both cohorts; group and family psychotherapy were employed much less frequently.

Table 3.9 details the average and median number of psychotherapy sessions among patients in the PTSD and depression cohorts who completed at least one ses-

Table 3.8
Percentage of Patients in the PTSD and Depression Cohorts Who Received Psychotherapy, 2013–2014

Treatment Modality	Percentage of PTSD Cohort	Percentage of Depression Cohort
Any psychotherapy	91.2	83.3
Individual psychotherapy	90.5	82.5
Group psychotherapy	26.9	19.5
Family psychotherapy	9.0	6.7

NOTES: Includes direct and purchased care. PTSD and depression cohorts are not mutually exclusive.

Table 3.9

Mean and Median Number of Psychotherapy Sessions in the Observation Period Among Those Who Received Psychotherapy, 2013–2014

Treatment Modality	PTSD Cohort Number of Sessions		Depression Cohort Number of Sessions	
	Mean (SD)	Median	Mean (SD)	Median
Any psychotherapy				
Any diagnosis	18.6 (17.4)	14	14.3 (14.8)	9
Cohort diagnosis[a]	14.6 (15.1)	9	8.6 (9.7)	5
Individual psychotherapy				
Any diagnosis	15.7 (13.7)	12	12.4 (12.1)	8
Cohort diagnosis[a]	12.8 (12.4)	9	8.1 (8.9)	5
Group psychotherapy				
Any diagnosis	12.2 (13.8)	7	9.8 (12.0)	5
Cohort diagnosis[a]	11.3 (12.8)	7	5.7 (7.6)	3
Family psychotherapy				
Any diagnosis	3.9 (5.4)	2	3.9 (5.0)	2
Cohort diagnosis[a]	3.3 (5.2)	2	3.1 (5.1)	1

NOTES: Includes direct and purchased care. Sessions were limited to one type of each therapy (e.g., individual, group, family) per date of service. SD = standard deviation. PTSD and depression cohorts are not mutually exclusive.

[a] The cohort diagnosis could have been recorded as a primary or secondary diagnosis.

sion. PTSD cohort patients received a median of 14 psychotherapy sessions (across treatment modalities) during the 12-month observation period, with a median of nine visits with a primary or secondary PTSD diagnosis. Members of the depression cohort received a median of nine psychotherapy sessions (across treatment modalities), with a median of five visits with a depression diagnosis (in any position). These results imply that patients were receiving psychotherapy related to their cohort diagnosis *and* other mental health conditions. Table 3.10 shows the frequency of psychotherapy sessions among patients in each cohort who received at least one session for any diagnosis. About 35 percent and 47 percent of PTSD and depression patients, respectively, attended one to eight psychotheraphy sessions during the 12-month observation window. Six percent of the PTSD cohort and 3 percent of the depression cohort attended more than 50 psychotherapy sessions.

Table 3.10
Percentage of Service Members, by Frequency of Psychotherapy Sessions Among Those Who Received Psychotherapy, 2013–2014

Cohort	Number of Sessions							Range of Sessions
	1–4	5–8	9–15	16–25	26–35	36–50	> 50	
PTSD cohort								
Any diagnosis	20.2	15.1	19.8	19.0	11.2	8.6	6.0	1–155
Cohort diagnosis[a]	30.0	17.0	18.6	16.3	8.9	5.8	3.5	1–146
Depression cohort								
Any diagnosis	28.3	18.6	20.0	16.0	8.3	5.6	3.2	1–168
Cohort diagnosis[a]	46.0	19.9	17.2	10.4	4.0	1.9	0.6	1–168

NOTES: Includes direct and purchased care. Sessions were limited to one type of each therapy (e.g., individual, group, family) per date of service. PTSD and depression cohorts are not mutually exclusive.
[a] The cohort diagnosis could have been recorded as a primary or secondary diagnosis.

Very few psychotherapy visits were delivered in primary care settings. Specifically, only about 4 percent (for PTSD or depression) of the total direct care cohort-related psychotherapy visits (of any duration) occurred in a primary care setting. Further, approximately 18 and 23 percent of all cohort-related psychotherapy visits (i.e., in any outpatient setting) for PTSD and depression, respectively, were coded as 30-minute sessions, with the remainder being longer than 30 minutes. The proportion of 30-minute sessions (versus longer sessions) for PTSD was 16 percent in primary care and 18 percent in behavioral health settings, while the proportion for depression was 32 percent in primary care and 23 percent in behavioral health.

Prescriptions for Psychotropic Medications Filled by Service Members in the PTSD and Depression Cohorts

Psychotropic medications have the ability to impact emotions and behavior and are grouped into five major classes: stimulants, antidepressants, antipsychotics, mood stabilizers, and antianxiety agents. In this section, we describe the number and types of prescribed psychotropic medications dispensed to patients in the PTSD and depression cohorts during the year-long observation period. Prazosin[6] is considered as a psychotropic class solely for the purpose of this report. Opioids are not included in the category of "other psychotropic medications" (which is limited to guanfacine and clonidine) but reported separately. The medication use described in this chapter is limited to medication dispensed for outpatient use.

First, we characterize the classes of psychotropic medications dispensed to patients in each cohort. We then detail the number of distinct prescription medications filled across and within each class of psychotropic medication.

Of those in the PTSD cohort, 78 percent filled an antidepressant prescription, and 57 percent filled a prescription for a hypnotic, sedative, or anxiolytic (including sleep medication, such as zolpidem) (Figure 3.7). Within the latter medication category, 33 percent of the PTSD cohort filled at least one prescription for a benzodiazepine (not shown). Approximately 33 percent of patients within the PTSD cohort filled a prescription for prazosin, and those in the PTSD cohort filled other medications with

Figure 3.7
Percentage of Patients in the PTSD Cohort Who Filled a Prescription for Psychotropic Medication (by Medication Class), 2013–2014

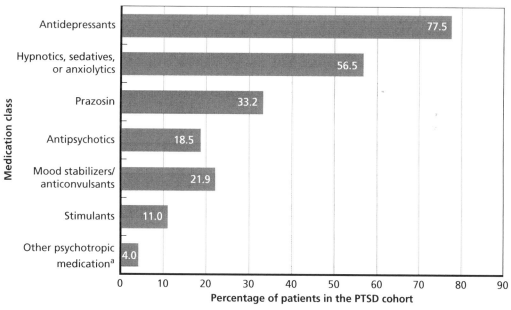

NOTE: Includes direct and purchased care.
[a] Includes guanfacine and clonidine.
RAND RR1542-3.7

---

[6]   Of those in the PTSD cohort treated with prazosin, a relatively small percentage had a concurrent diagnosis of hypertension (22.9 percent) or benign prostatic hyperplasia (1.5 percent), suggesting that in the majority of cases, the medication was used for its psychotropic effects.

the frequency indicated: antipsychotic (19 percent), mood stabilizer/anticonvulsant (22 percent), stimulant (11 percent), and other psychotropic medication (4 percent). In addition to the medication classes presented here, 57 percent of the PTSD cohort filled at least one prescription for an opioid (not shown).

Psychotropic medications filled by service members in the depression cohort are shown in Figure 3.8. Nearly four-fifths (79 percent) of the depression cohort filled a prescription for an antidepressant, and almost half of the cohort (46 percent) filled a prescription for a hypnotic, sedative, or anxiolytic, including 25 percent of the depression cohort filling a prescription for a benzodiazepine (not shown). Similar to the PTSD cohort, a smaller percentage of depression cohort patients filled other types of prescriptions: mood stabilizer/anticonvulsant (16 percent), and other psychotropic medication (2 percent). In addition, 50 percent of the depression cohort filled at least one prescription for an opioid (not shown).

These findings demonstrate that many service members in the PTSD and depression cohorts received multiple types of psychotropic medications. Furthermore, in the two cohorts, 50 percent or more filled a prescription for an opioid, and 25 to 33 percent filled a prescription for a benzodiazepine. In interpreting these results it is important to note there is considerable overlap between the PTSD and depression cohorts; a sizable

Figure 3.8
Percentage of Patients in the Depression Cohort Who Filled a Prescription for Psychotropic Medication (by Medication Class), 2013–2014

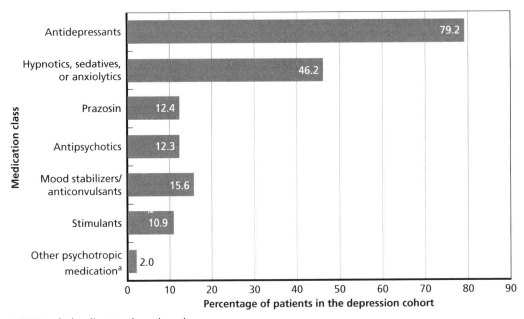

NOTE: Includes direct and purchased care.
a Includes guanfacine and clonidine.
RAND RR1542-3.8

percentage of service members in the PTSD cohort are also in the depression cohort, and vice versa. Secondly, it is important to note that these results are based on psychotropic prescriptions filled over the entire 12-month observation period. Further data analysis would be needed to explore longitudinal patterns of medication use, highlight overlap in medication regimens, examine concurrent use of nonpsychotropic medications, and assess the appropriateness of the regimens prescribed.

Lastly, we describe the number of psychotropic medications filled by service members in the PTSD and depression cohorts. We first present the number of distinct medications filled across and within each class of psychotropic medication. Then, we examine the number of different classes of prescriptions for psychotropic medications filled by the patients in each cohort.

Of service members in the PTSD cohort, 86 percent received at least one psychotropic medication, while the remaining 14 percent did not (Table 3.11). Approximately 45 percent received four or more psychotropic medications. Of service members in the depression cohort, 85 percent received at least one psychotropic medication, while the remaining 15 percent did not (Table 3.12). Approximately one third of patients (32 percent) received four or more psychotropic medications. Tables 3.11 and 3.12 also describe the proportion of cohort members who filled prescriptions for different medications within the aforementioned medication classes. Information about prescriptions by class provides further insight regarding the patterns of psychotropic pharmaco-

Table 3.11
Percentage of Patients in the PTSD Cohort Who Filled Prescriptions for Psychotropic Medications, 2013–2014

Class of Medication	Number of Psychotropic Medications						
	0	1	2	3	4–6	7–10	11 or more
Psychotropic, from all classes	14.4	12.3	14.0	14.5	29.6	12.9	2.4
Antidepressants	22.5	28.9	25.6	13.9	8.8	0.2	0
Antipsychotics	81.5	14.7	3.0	0.7	0.2	0	0
Hypnotics, sedatives, or anxiolytics	43.5	30.7	15.3	7.0	3.4	< 0.1	0
Stimulants	89.0	9.1	1.7	0.2	< 0.1	0	—
Mood stabilizers/ anticonvulsants	78.1	19.3	2.3	0.3	< 0.1	—	—
Other psychotropic medication [a]	96.0	4.0	< 0.1	—	—	—	—
Prazosin	66.8	33.2	—	—	—	—	—

NOTE: Includes direct and purchased care.

[a] Includes guanfacine and clonidine.

Table 3.12
Percentage of Patients in the Depression Cohort Who Filled Prescriptions for Psychotropic Medications, 2013–2014

Class of Medication	Number of Psychotropic Medications						
	0	1	2	3	4–6	7–10	11 or more
Psychotropic, from all classes	14.6	20.2	19.0	14.6	22.5	7.7	1.3
Antidepressants	20.8	35.5	25.1	11.7	6.7	0.2	0
Antipsychotics	87.7	9.8	2.1	0.4	0.1	0	0
Hypnotics, sedatives, or anxiolytics	53.8	27.6	12.0	4.5	2.0	< 0.1	0
Stimulants	89.1	9.0	1.6	0.3	< 0.1	0	—
Mood stabilizers/anticonvulsants	84.4	13.9	1.5	0.2	< 0.1	—	—
Other psychotropic medication [a]	98.0	2.0	< 0.1	—	—	—	—
Prazosin	87.6	12.4	—	—	—	—	—

NOTE: Includes direct and purchased care.

[a] Includes guanfacine and clonidine.

therapy in the two cohorts and highlights the complex pharmacologic regimens they were prescribed. A large percentage of the PTSD and depression cohorts filled prescriptions for more than one psychotropic medication within the same class. For example, approximately 49 percent of patients in the PTSD cohort and 44 percent of patients in the depression cohort filled prescriptions for two or more antidepressants during the observation period. Similar examples can be found in most of the medication classes presented. Most of these are service members with prescriptions for two or three psychotropic medications within the same class; filling prescriptions for more than three drugs within a single class is much less common for all classes except antidepressants. Again, these analyses do not examine the appropriateness of the psychotropic medicines prescribed, nor do they consider the simultaneous use of nonpsychotropic medications. More extensive and detailed analytical approaches are required to adequately address these complex patterns of pharmacotherapy.

The numbers of psychotropic medication classes for which PTSD and depression cohort patients filled prescriptions during the observation period are shown in Figures 3.9 and 3.10. Between 14 and 15 percent of each cohort did not fill any prescriptions for psychotropic medications. Nearly one-fifth of the PTSD cohort (18 percent) and approximately one-third of the depression cohort (31 percent) filled prescriptions from only one psychotropic medication class. About a quarter of the PTSD cohort and 29 percent of the depression cohort filled prescriptions from two different classes. Forty-two percent of the PTSD cohort and 26 percent of the depression cohort filled prescriptions from three or more classes of psychotropic medications. These findings indi-

Figure 3.9
Percentage of Patients in the PTSD Cohort Who
Filled a Prescription from Different Psychotropic
Medication Classes, 2013–2014

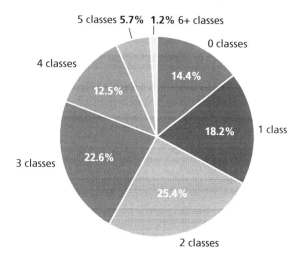

NOTE: Includes direct and purchased care.
RAND RR1542-3.9

Figure 3.10
Percentage of Patients in the Depression Cohort
Who Filled a Prescription from Different
Psychotropic Medication Classes, 2013–2014

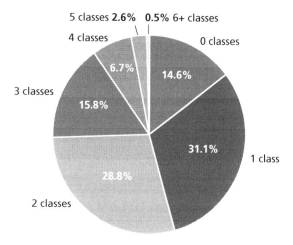

NOTE: Includes direct and purchased care.
RAND RR1542-3.10

cate that a substantial percentage of patients fill prescriptions for multiple psychotropic medications. Given that such regimens likely increase the complexity of these service members' care, this underscores the need for prescribing providers to carefully manage psychotropic pharmacotherapy.

Summary

In this chapter, we presented a detailed characterization of the service members in the PTSD and depression cohorts and the care they received over their one-year observation period. The analyses in this chapter do not include examination of quality measures but rather describe the characteristics and patterns of care among service members in these two cohorts. We provided information about their demographic and military service characteristics, the settings in which they received health care services, the type of services, and the providers who treated them. Lastly, we described the various types of assessments and treatments these service members received, including behavioral interventions and psychotropic medications. Our results are summarized here.

In both the PTSD and depression cohorts, the majority of active-component service members were soldiers, enlisted (versus officer), and had experienced at least one deployment. Cohort members were also more likely to be male, white, married, and under 35 years of age. Although the two cohorts had similar demographic and service characteristics, a higher proportion of individuals in the depression cohort were female, never married, under 25 years of age, and never deployed. It is important to note that a substantial number of patients were in *both* the PTSD and depression cohorts. Furthermore, more than half of patients in the PTSD cohort had a diagnosis of depression, and more than a quarter of those in the depression cohort received a PTSD diagnosis during the 12 month observation period.

The majority of patients in both the PTSD and depression cohorts received care for their cohort diagnosis solely at MTFs, and a small percentage of each cohort utilized only purchased care. A moderate proportion of patients in each cohort received both direct and purchased care. Individuals in both cohorts received care for conditions not associated with their cohort diagnosis (PTSD or depression). Nearly 60 percent of all primary diagnoses were coded for non-PH diagnoses, although our analyses did not examine the specific non–mental health conditions for which cohort members received care. Adjustment disorders, anxiety disorders, and sleep disorders or symptoms were the most prevalent co-occurring PH disorders in the two cohorts. Although patients in both the PTSD and depression cohorts saw a wide range of providers for care associated with their cohort diagnosis, they most commonly visited primary care and mental health care providers (specifically psychiatrists, clinical psychologists, and social workers). These findings indicate that service members with PTSD or depression may be seen by multiple providers in both primary and specialty care settings. Accordingly, it is critical that future analyses carefully examine these patterns of health care utilization across both psychological health and non-psychological health conditions to inform care coordination and management efforts for these patients. In both cohorts, most patients received at least some care associated with their cohort diagnosis in a mental health care setting. It appeared that service members in the PTSD cohort were more likely to be seen in specialty care settings and by specialty care providers than those in the depression cohort, although these cohort comparisons are challenging due to the overlap in the cohorts. Approximately 20 percent of patients in each cohort had at least one inpatient stay (for any diagnosis), and 14 to 15 percent of the cohorts had an inpatient stay related to their cohort condition.

While more than two-thirds of patients in both cohorts received psychiatric diagnostic evaluation or psychological testing, other methods of testing and assessment, such as neuropsychological testing and health and behavior assessment, were less commonly used. A large percentage of both the PTSD cohort (91 percent) and the depression cohort (83 percent) received at least one psychotherapy visit (individual, group, or family therapy). Additionally, for both cohorts, individual therapy was received most often, and family therapy was received least frequently. PTSD cohort patients who received psychotherapy had a median of 14 visits over the observation period (across therapy modalities), with a median of nine visits associated with a PTSD diagnosis code (in either the primary or secondary position). Individuals in the depression cohort received a median of nine psychotherapy visits, with a median of five sessions with a depression diagnosis code in any position. Among patients who received psychotherapy for any diagnosis, 20 percent of both the PTSD and depression cohorts had between nine and 15 sessions during the observation period. A larger percentage of the PTSD cohort had 16 or more sessions than did the depression cohort (45 and 33 percent, respectively). While there is likely variation at the individual patient level in the number of visits received, these findings suggest that some of the patients are receiving a number of therapy sessions that is consistent with clinical guidelines. Approximately 6 percent of the PTSD cohort and 3 percent of the depression cohort had over 50 psychotherapy visits.

Approximately 86 percent of each cohort filled at least one prescription for a psychotropic medication. In both cohorts, antidepressants were the most common class of psychotropic medicine dispensed, while stimulants were the least. Patients in the PTSD and depression cohorts often filled prescriptions for more than one psychotropic medication, both across and within medication classes. More than a quarter of each cohort had prescriptions from two different classes, while 42 percent of the PTSD cohort and 26 percent of the depression cohort filled prescriptions from three or more classes of psychotropic medications. Furthermore, a sizable percentage of patients in both cohorts filled prescriptions for two or medications within the same psychotropic class. These results indicate that patients in both cohorts receive a wide range of psychotropic medications, and, given this complexity, providers should exercise caution in managing patients' treatment. Also, 33 percent of PTSD patients and 25 percent of depression patients filled a prescription for a benzodiazepine, and slightly more than half of both cohorts filled a prescription for an opioid.

While the descriptive utilization data described in this chapter do not explicitly examine the quality of care, several findings stand out and suggest priorities for more in-depth evaluation of quality. First, the high utilization for both medical and psychological conditions combined with the high number of different providers raise questions about the extent of coordination versus fragmentation of care for all the care these service members received. Second, the high number of psychotherapy visits received by members of these cohorts suggests that the MHS may be more successful than the civilian sector in engaging patients with PTSD or depression in psychosocial interventions. A study of psychotherapy utilization among privately insured patients found that PTSD patients received a mean of 12.6 therapy visits (compared with a mean of 18.6 in our PTSD cohort), while MDD patients received a mean of 9.9 visits (compared with a mean of 14.3 in our depression cohort) (Harpaz-Rotem, Libby, and Rosenheck, 2012). Examination of the reasons for this success should be quite informative to future efforts. Third, a majority of members of both cohorts received multiple psychotropic medications over the course of the observation year, both within and across classes of these medications (and a significant number received opioid medications as well). It should be noted that the medications discussed in this chapter were dispensed in addition to any nonpsychotropic medications not included in these analyses. Further examination is necessary to characterize the nature and appropriateness of these complex patterns of pharmacologic care. For example, additional analyses could examine the degree to which psychotropic medications are concurrent, rather than sequential, and potential risks associated with concurrent prescribing.

CHAPTER FOUR

Quality of Care for PTSD

PTSD Quality Measure Scores, 2013–2014

In this chapter, we present the results of analyses **focused on the outpatient care** provided to active-component service members with a diagnosis of PTSD using the quality measures based on administrative data, MRR, and symptom questionnaire data collected through the BHDP. These measures are outlined in Chapters One and Two, and technical specifications are detailed extensively in Appendix A.[1] **The administrative data measures represent outpatient care provided in both direct care and purchased care settings. We analyzed outpatient medical record data for a smaller sample of active-component service members who received only direct care provided by MTFs. The measures based on symptom questionnaire data represent active-component service members in the Army with direct care only and visits to behavioral health specialty care.** Table 4.1 shows the characteristics of the service members in the PTSD cohort, in the MRR sample for PTSD, and in the symptom questionnaire sample for PTSD. Many characteristics of the three groups are similar. However, those in the MRR sample and the group with symptom questionnaires used to determine quality measure scores were limited to service members who received direct care only. The symptom questionnaire group was also limited to those in the Army. The PTSD MRR sample differed from the other two because it was stratified to include a larger proportion of service members beginning an NTE (i.e., 57 percent in the MRR sample; 19 percent in the cohort; 22 percent in the symptom questionnaire sample). Utilization of care for the PTSD MRR sample was also much lower than for the other two, perhaps a reflection of the higher proportion of NTEs. The MRR and symptom questionnaire samples both had lower utilization than the cohort, perhaps reflecting the limitation of those samples to service members with direct care only. The overlap among the three groups is shown in Figure 4.1. The care provided to each service member with a PTSD diagnosis should be consistent with the PTSD guidelines, as assessed by the PTSD quality measures, even among those who also have a diagnosis of depression.

---

[1] Appendixes for this report are available online: http://www.rand.org/pubs/research_reports/RR1542.html.

Table 4.1
Characteristics of Service Members with PTSD in the Cohort, MRR Sample, and with Symptom Questionnaire Data Used to Calculate Quality Measure Scores

Characteristic	Cohort % (N)	MRR Sample % (N)	Symptom Questionnaire % (N)
Total	100 (14,654)	100 (400)	100 (2,583)
Gender			
Female	19.2 (2,819)	17.5 (70)	13.2 (342)
Race/ethnicity			
American Indian/Alaskan native	1.5 (213)	1.8 (7)	1.0 (25)
Asian/Pacific Islander	4.8 (700)	5.5 (22)	6.4 (165)
Black, non-Hispanic	20.0 (2,927)	17.3 (69)	23.0 (595)
White, non-Hispanic	58.6 (8,581)	57.8 (231)	55.1 (1,423)
Hispanic	13.1 (1,924)	15.3 (61)	13.6 (351)
Other	2.1 (309)	2.5 (10)	0.9 (24)
Age			
18–24	14.8 (2,175)	17.3 (69)	12.0 (311)
25–34	45.3 (6,644)	47.3 (189)	46.4 (1,198)
35–44	33.8 (4,954)	31.0 (124)	35.3 (911)
45 and over	6.0 (881)	4.5 (18)	6.3 (163)
Service			
Army	68.6 (10,045)	59.3 (237)	100 (2,583)
Air Force	11.5 (1,692)	10.3 (41)	NA
Marine Corps	10.5 (1,543)	15.0 (60)	NA
Navy	8.5 (1,245)	15.5 (62)	NA
Coast Guard	0.9 (129)	NA	NA
Region			
North	21.1 (3,096)	17.0 (68)	11.3 (291)
South	34.3 (5,019)	25.0 (100)	30.9 (799)
West	32.1 (4,705)	40.0 (160)	31.4 (811)
Overseas	10.4 (1,518)	18.0 (72)	24.5 (633)
Unknown	2.2 (316)	NA	1.9 (49)

Table 4.1—Continued

Characteristic	Cohort % (N)	MRR Sample % (N)	Symptom Questionnaire % (N)
Never deployed[a]	10.1 (1,478)	11.5 (46)	5.3 (137)
Have an NTE	19.1 (2,793)	57.3 (229)	21.6 (557)
Direct care only	35.0 (5,134)	100 (400)	100 (2,583)
Received any acute inpatient care	21.3 (3,115)	5.8 (23)	10.1 (262)
Received any inpatient care with a primary mental health discharge diagnosis	13.0 (1,908)	2.3 (9)	4.3 (112)
Median outpatient encounters for any diagnosis (for those with at least one)	40	24	30
Median outpatient encounters with a primary mental health diagnosis (for those with at least one)	17	10	13

NOTE: MRR = medical record review.

[a] Based on data from September 2001 through March 2015

Figure 4.1
Three Sources for PTSD Measure Denominators

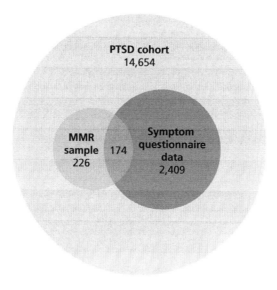

In the following sections, we present the results of our evaluation of care for PTSD. Each quality measure focuses on the subset of patients who met the eligibility requirements as specified in the measure denominator. Measure denominators have specifications that not all patients will meet, such as starting a new medication, having a particular type of health care encounter, or starting a new treatment episode. As a result, 39 percent of the PTSD cohort was included in at least one administrative data measure denominator, 93 percent of the MRR sample in at least one MRR data measure, and 93 percent of the symptom questionnaire group was included in at least one measure using symptom questionnaire data. We present results for the MHS as a whole, including comparative results from other health care systems, and then present variations by service branch and TRICARE region for measures based on administrative data.

Assessment: Symptom Severity and Comorbidity

Four measures focus on assessments addressing symptom severity and comorbidity for patients with a new treatment episode of PTSD. The measure titles, statements, numerators, and denominators are shown in Table 4.2.

These measures were adapted from the VHA Mental Health Program Evaluation (Farmer et al., 2010; Watkins et al., 2011). Information about symptom severity and comorbidity are necessary to guide the development of an appropriate treatment plan.

Table 4.2
PTSD Assessment Measures: Symptom Severity and Comorbidity

Measure Title	Measure Statement	Numerator	Denominator
Baseline symptom assessment with the PCL [PTSD-A1]	Percentage of PTSD patients with an NTE with assessment of symptoms with the PCL within 30 days	Patients with an assessment of symptoms with the PCL within 30 days	PTSD patients with an NTE
Assessment for depression [PTSD-A2]	Percentage of PTSD patients with an NTE assessed for depression within 30 days	Patients with an assessment for depression within 30 days	PTSD patients with an NTE
Assessment for suicide risk [PTSD-A3]	Percentage of PTSD patients with an NTE assessed for suicide risk at the same visit	Patients with an assessment for suicide risk at the same visit	PTSD patients with an NTE
Assessment for recent substance use [PTSD-A4]	Percentage of PTSD patients with an NTE assessed for recent substance use within 30 days	Patients with an assessment for recent substance use within 30 days	PTSD patients with an NTE

NOTE: NTE = new treatment episode.

Baseline Symptom Assessment with the PCL [PTSD-A1]. Although the VHA evaluation accepted using any one of many standardized tools and structured interviews for baseline PTSD symptom assessment, we recommend the use of the PCL to establish an objective, baseline score and means for monitoring the patient's response to treatment over time. The PCL is a 17-item measure reflecting DSM-IV self-reported symptoms of PTSD (Weathers et al., 2013). The PCL was also incorporated into this measure because of its recommended use by the MHS (DoD, 2014e).[2] The VA/DoD CPGs (VA and DoD, 2010) cite evidence supporting thorough assessment of PTSD symptoms for patients in both primary and mental health specialty care settings (Lagomasino, Daly, and Stoudemire, 1999; Williams and Shepherd, 2000). Harding et al. (2011) make the case for measurement-based care as the standard for psychiatric practice to align with physical health care.

Assessments for Depression [PTSD-A2] and Recent Substance Use [PTSD-A4]. The VA/DoD CPGs (VA and DoD, 2010) also recommend assessing the newly diagnosed PTSD patient for a range of psychiatric comorbidities, including depression and substance use in order to plan treatment accordingly and to limit factors that may be caused by and/or exacerbate the PTSD symptoms. The assessment measures for screening for depression (PTSD-A2) and substance use (PTSD-A4) incorporate the use of either a standardized tool or an informal assessment within 30 days of diagnosis. The 30-day time frame includes assessments that may have been done just prior to or shortly after the diagnosis of the condition.

Assessment for Suicide Risk [PTSD-A3]. The CPGs also recommend assessing the patient with PTSD for safety and risk to self and others. It is notable that DoD has increased attention on preventing suicide among service members. In 2008, the age-adjusted suicide rate in active-component service members exceeded that in civilians, 20.2 compared with 19.2, respectively (VA and DoD, 2013). In 2014 among active-component service members across all service branches, the suicide rate was 19.9 per 100,000 (DoD, 2016). The 2014 suicide rate varied by branch of service, with Army having the highest rate (23.8 per 100,000) followed by Air Force (18.5 per 100,000), Marine Corps (17.9 per 100,000), and Navy (16.3 per 100,000). The measure addressing assessment for suicide risk (PTSD-A3) allows for the use of a standardized tool or informal assessment but is required to be done at the same visit that started the NTE. If the screen was positive for suicidal ideation (SI), the measure required a documented assessment for plan and access to lethal means (if not hospitalized).

---

[2]   The diagnostic criteria for PTSD were updated in the 2013 revision of *Diagnostic and Statistical Manual of Mental Disorders*, 5th ed. (DSM-5) (American Psychiatric Association, 2013). A revised version of the PCL (PCL-5) reflects these changes (Weathers et al., 2013). It will be important to track the future use of this instrument and update measure-scoring protocols accordingly.

Table 4.3
PTSD Measure Scores Related to Assessment of Symptom Severity and Comorbidity, 2013–2014

Measure	Numerator[a]	Denominator[b]	Measure Score
Percentage of PTSD patients in an NTE with assessment of symptoms with the PCL[c] [PTSD-A1]	107	229	46.7%
Percentage of PTSD patients in an NTE assessed for depression [PTSD-A2]	215	229	93.9%
Percentage of PTSD patients in an NTE assessed for suicide risk [PTSD-A3]	220	229	96.1%
Percentage of PTSD patients in an NTE assessed for recent substance use [PTSD-A4]	213	229	93.0%

[a] Based on medical record data; direct care only.

[b] Based on administrative data; direct care only.

[c] Unlike other measures utilizing the PCL (T1, T10, and 12) which were scored using the BHDP, measure PTSD-A1 numerator was scored using data from the medical record, since abstractors were collecting data for the other three assessments (PTSD A2, A3, and A4). While BHDP PCL scores are intended to be entered into the medical record, this may not happen in every instance. Therefore, a limitation of the data used for this measure is that a score entered within 30 days of the NTE into the BHDP would have been missed if not also entered into the medical record. Prior to curtailing data collection, we looked at a small sample of patients and compared scores from the BHDP data to scores collected from the medical record. At that point in time, neither source appeared to be superior. in that while some scores were identical in the two sources, others were missing from either source with similar frequency.

Measure Results

Measure score results for the four assessment measures are shown in Table 4.3. Approximately 47 percent of PTSD patients in a new treatment episode in the MRR sample were assessed with the PCL at the same visit as the start of the NTE or within 30 days prior or 30 days after that visit (PTSD-A1). Other NTE assessments were performed more frequently: depression, 94 percent; suicide risk, 96 percent; and recent substance use (either alcohol or drugs), 93 percent. Of the 215 patients screened for depression (PTSD-A2), 126 patients (58.6 percent) were screened informally, and 89 patients (41.4 percent) were screened with a standardized tool, most often the PHQ-2 or PHQ-9.

Screening for suicide risk (PTSD-A3) was most often completed with an informal assessment, rather than use of a standardized tool. Of the 220 patients assessed for SI on the date of diagnosis, a standardized tool was used in 37 patients (16.8 percent). For almost all of these patients, the provider used the single suicide item from the PHQ-9. Of the patients who did not meet the criteria for this measure, all nine had no documented evidence of a screen for SI. Of the small number of patients with a positive screen for SI identified in this measure, all passed based on documentation that included an assessment for presence or absence of a suicide plan and a restriction of lethal means discussion.

When screening for recent substance use (PTSD-A4), providers screened 80 percent of patients for recent alcohol use and 83.4 percent of patients for recent drug use. Providers most often used informal screens (69.9 percent for alcohol and 99 percent for drug use). When a standardized tool was used to screen for alcohol use, the tool of choice was the Alcohol Use Disorders Identification Test–Consumption (AUDIT-C) (72.7 percent) or the full AUDIT (23.6 percent) (Saunders et al., 1993).

Comparative Results from Other Sources

Baseline Symptom Assessment with the PCL [PTSD-A1]. One study of veterans with a new treatment episode for PTSD in FY 2007 found that 5.6 percent had an assessment of PTSD symptoms with a standardized instrument or structured interview within the first 30 days within the VHA system of care (Farmer et al., 2010). While the patients included in our study are active-component service members, those in the Farmer et al. (2010) evaluation were veterans. Furthermore, our study was conducted after recent DoD endorsement of the PCL as the preferred outcomes measure for PTSD (DoD, 2013), and at the start of the expansion of the BHDP usage across all Army MTFs (Committee on the Assessment of Ongoing Efforts in the Treatment of Posttraumatic Stress Disorder, 2014). While the measure score of 46.7 percent in our study indicates room for improvement, it demonstrates higher use than the earlier VA evaluation. This score is likely to increase in the future with the recommended regular use of the PCL to monitor patient progress (DoD 2014e). While the initial assessment is important as a baseline clinical measure, longitudinal assessment as part of a Measurement-Based Care strategy would be valuable.

Assessment for Depression [PTSD-A2]. An evaluation of VHA mental health services (Farmer et al., 2010) found 85.6 percent of veterans in a PTSD cohort were assessed for depression within the first 30 days of a PTSD NTE. Our study found 93.9 percent of service members in the sample of PTSD patients starting an NTE were assessed for depression within 30 days. This measure score is relatively high and suggests that MHS performs well at ensuring that active-component service members diagnosed with PTSD are evaluated for depression as an additional psychological comorbidity.

Assessment for Suicide Risk [PTSD-A3]. Comparative data for this finding stems from analyses of suicide risk assessments among veteran populations in the United States. The rate of suicide risk assessment was 81.8 percent for veterans who received services from the VHA in FY 2007 for at least one of the following diagnoses: schizophrenia, bipolar I disorder, PTSD, major depression, or substance use disorders (Farmer et al., 2010). That metric represented the percentage of veterans in the study who had at least one screen for SI in the medical record during the 12-month measurement period. When restricted to veterans with one of the aforementioned diagnoses who received specialty mental health care, the measure score increased to 93.1 percent (Farmer et al., 2010). The high rate of suicide risk assessment (96.1 percent) among active service members with a new treatment episode of PTSD in this study suggests that MHS has successfully integrated evaluations for suicide risk as a routine aspect of its psychological health care delivery system for PTSD.

Assessment for Recent Substance Use [PTSD-A4]. The percentage with substance use assessment among veterans across five diagnostic cohorts (schizophrenia, bipolar I disorder, PTSD, major depression, or substance use disorder) within 30 days of an NTE in the VHA health system was 71.8 percent (Farmer et al., 2010). A review of VA outpatient medical records from 2005 across 21 VHA networks showed 93 percent of patients were screened for alcohol misuse (Bradley et al., 2006). Comparison of these findings with our study shows MHS screening rates for substance use among active-component service members newly diagnosed with PTSD (93.0 percent) to be on par with VHA measure scores for alcohol misuse screening among veterans.

Treatment: Follow-up for Suicidal Ideation

This measure focuses on the assessment and treatment of service members with PTSD who presented with or had a positive screen for suicidal ideation (Table 4.4).

Measure Rationale and Overview

A similar follow-up measure was used in the VHA Mental Health Program Evaluation (Farmer et al., 2010; Watkins et al., 2011). That measure has been significantly modified here based on the *VA/DoD Clinical Practice Guideline for Assessment and Management of Patients at Risk for Suicide* (VA and DoD, 2013). The CPG specifies that the recommended course of treatment for SI be tied to a clinical judgment of whether the acute risk for suicide is low, intermediate, or high. That acute risk status judgment (low, intermediate, high) is then mapped onto several possible clinical responses. When acute risk status is low, the provider can choose to consult with a behavioral health provider, or address the safety issues and treat the presenting problems without such a consult. When acute risk status is intermediate, the minimum recommendations are to limit access to lethal means, conduct a complete behavioral evaluation (or refer to a behav-

Table 4.4
PTSD Treatment Measures: Follow-up for Suicidal Ideation, 2013–2014

Measure Title	Measure Statement	Numerator	Denominator
Appropriate follow-up for endorsed suicidal ideation [PTSD-T3]	Percentage of patient contacts of PTSD patients with SI with appropriate follow-up (PTSD-T3)	Patients with appropriate follow-up on the same day that the suicidal ideation was documented	PTSD patient visit where positive suicidal ideation was documented

ioral health provider to do so), and determine an appropriate referral. When acute risk status is high, the guidelines recommend maintenance of direct observational control of the patient and transfer to an emergency care setting for hospitalization.

We had planned to limit application of the suicidal ideation follow-up measure (PTSD-T3) to a smaller subset of patients whose providers had assessed and documented the patient's level of suicide risk as low, intermediate, or high. The level of risk, based on other assessments of comorbid risk and supportive factors, determined the minimum interventions required for appropriate care for this measure. However, the number of PTSD patients with SI with a documented high/intermediate/low risk level was just 15. This may well reflect the very recent release of the suicide risk CPG at the time of data collection, which may not have allowed enough time for general implementation into the MTFs. Therefore, we opted to apply a single minimal level of required care, for all 24 patients with SI, that included (for patients not hospitalized) three required elements: (1) an assessment for plan and access to lethal means, (2) a referral or appointment for follow-up, and (3) a discussion of limitation of access to lethal means or documentation that the access assessment was negative. These requirements follow the recommendations in the CPG's decisionmaking Algorithm A for low-risk patients (VA and DoD, 2013). The care assessed for this measure was limited to that related to the first episode of suicidal ideation (SI) noted in the record during the measurement period.[3] Appropriate care needed to have been provided on the same day that the SI was documented.

Measure Results

During medical record review, abstractors identified 24 PTSD patients with at least one occurrence of suicidal ideation. For 23 (95.8 percent) of these patients, the provider who documented the positive SI was a behavioral health provider. Among the 24 patients with positive SI, 13 (54.2 percent) had documentation of all three elements of appropriate care on the same day when SI was documented (Table 4.5). Not meeting the criteria for this measure was most often related to not addressing lethal means (10 patients); that is, either there was no documented assessment of access to lethal means,

Table 4.5
PTSD Measure Score for Follow-up of Suicidal Ideation, 2013–2014

Measure	Numerator[a]	Denominator[a]	Measure Score
Percentage of patient contacts of PTSD patients with SI with appropriate follow-up (PTSD-T3)	13	24	54.2%

[a] Based on medical record data; direct care only.

---

[3]   The time period for identifying SI was initially the entire 12 months of the measurement period, but this was later reduced during the medical record abstraction to the first six months due to time constraints. See Chapter Two, Methods.

Table 4.6
Risk Factor Assessments of Service Members with PTSD Performed on the Same Day the Suicidal Ideation Was Documented

Assessed for presence or absence of:[a]	Patients with positive SI (n = 24) % (N)
SI persistence	95.8 (23)
Intent	95.8 (23)
Plan	91.7 (22)
Access to means	70.8 (17)
Suicide risk level assigned as high, intermediate, or low	62.5 (15)
Recent suicidal behavior	50.0 (12)
Recent suicide attempt	87.5 (21)
History of prior attempt	83.3 (20)
Recent substance use	83.3 (20)
History of prior substance use	70.8 (17)

NOTE: SI = suicidal ideation.

[a] Based on medical record data; direct care only.

or the provider documented access to lethal means but did not document a discussion with the patient on how to limit access to those means.

We also summarized the types and frequencies of suicide-related assessments performed at the visit where the SI was noted for all 24 patients with positive SI (Table 4.6.). These assessments represent indicators of risk and contributing factors from the CPG that could assist the provider in determining the overall level of the patient's suicide risk and, thereby, guide the provision of appropriate care (VA and DoD, 2013). Almost all patients (95.8 percent) were assessed for the persistence of the SI (i.e., constant, intermittent, or present in the past two weeks) and the level of the patient's intent (i.e., presence or absence of intention to act on the SI). A large proportion (91.7 percent) was also assessed for the presence of a suicide plan. Fewer patients (70.8 percent) were assessed for access to means to carry out a suicide. When limited to patients who were not hospitalized, this proportion falls to 61.1 percent. Overall, the level of suicide risk was classified as high, intermediate, or low for 62.5 percent. Half of those with SI had documented information about the presence or absence of recent suicidal behavior. Assessments for recent or prior suicide attempts were conducted in 83 to 88 percent of patients. Providers documented assessments for recent and prior substance use for 71 to 83 percent of patients.

We also summarized interventions provided in treating the 24 patients with SI at the time of the visit (Table 4.7). All of the patients had a behavioral health consult and six (25 percent) of the 24 patients were hospitalized. For those not hospitalized,

Table 4.7
Interventions for Service Members with PTSD on the Same Day the Suicidal ideation Was Documented

Intervention	Patients with positive SI (n = 24) % (N)
Hospitalized[a]	25.0 (6)
Assessed by behavioral health[a]	100 (24)
For those not hospitalized:	*(n=18)*
Lethal means discussion or documented negative assessment for access to means[a]	44.4 (8)
Referral to behavioral health or to the same provider[a]	94.4 (17)
Next visit with any provider occurred within:[b]	
1 week	66.7 (12)
2–3 weeks	33.3 (6)
Next visit with a behavioral health provider occurred within:[b]	
1 week	55.6 (10)
2–3 weeks	44.4 (8)

[a] Based on medical record data; direct care only.

[b] Based on administrative data; direct care only.

44.4 percent had documentation of counseling about limiting access to lethal means or a negative assessment for access to means. Almost all patients (94.4 percent) were given a referral to a behavioral health provider and/or were instructed to follow up with the same provider at the conclusion of the visit. Based on administrative data, all 18 patients not hospitalized subsequently had a visit with any type of provider within three weeks, with over half (66.7 percent) being seen within one week. Mental health providers saw most patients within one week and all within three weeks.

Comparative Results from Other Sources

Appropriate Follow-up for Endorsed Suicidal Ideation [PTSD-T3]. We found limited comparative data for this measure. Of veterans who received VHA care in FY 2007 for at least one of five psychological disorders (schizophrenia, bipolar I disorder, PTSD, major depression, or substance use disorder), 96.4 percent received appropriate follow-up for suicidal ideation on the same date the SI was documented (Farmer et al., 2010). Appropriateness of follow-up in that study was determined by the abstractor's assessment of the follow-up documented in the medical record. This included assessment for intent, plan, and means, and interventions applied (in the absence of hospitalization), such as discussion of safety, provision of a list of appropriate resources, and appointment for follow-up. Discretion was left to the abstractor to determine whether the follow-up was appropriate based on documented data about the patient in the medical record. In this study, abstractors collected data elements about the assessments and follow-up care, and the appropriateness of follow-up was determined in analysis according to the requirements noted earlier.

The results presented in the current study are based on a small sample of patients and on a CPG for suicide risk management that had only recently been published (June 2013). The 18-month window for this study included a cohort selection window from January through June 2013, and observation of care in the subsequent 12 months that could have continued as long as through June of 2014. Therefore, there may have been only limited uptake of the CPG during the time we observed care. The assessment and management of suicide risk is an extremely important and complex clinical entity. We made a concerted effort to include essential items drawn from the CPGs (particularly those cited as important for determining the level of suicide risk and appropriate action in Table 1, p. 48 of the CPG [VA and DoD, 2013]) and had experts from DoD and VA review the content of our data collection tool. While the sample is small, our results suggest that appropriate follow-up for suicide risk should be a high-priority target for improvement, which could be geared toward increasing discussion of lethal means. Since this study was initiated, a Safety Plan Worksheet VA, 2014) was added to the 2013 CPG for suicide risk management; it incorporates limitation of access to lethal means. Generalized use of this tool could facilitate improved scores for this measure.

Treatment: Medication Management

The two measures that address medication management consider the duration of a newly prescribed SSRI/SNRI for patients with PTSD and a follow-up evaluation in the 30 days following dispensing of the medication (Table 4.8).

Table 4.8
PTSD Treatment Measures: Medication Management, 2013–2014

Measure Title	Measure Statement	Numerator	Denominator
Duration of new SSRI/SNRI treatment [PTSD-T5]	Percentage of PTSD patients with a newly prescribed SSRI/SNRI for ≥ 60 days	PTSD patients who receive a newly prescribed SSRI/SNRI for ≥ 60 days	Patients with PTSD who fill a new prescription for an SSRI/SNRI
Follow-up of new prescription for SSRI/SNRI [PTSD-T6]	Percentage of PTSD patients newly prescribed an SSRI/SNRI with follow-up visit within 30 days	PTSD patients who have a follow-up visit within 30 days a new prescription for a SSRI/SNRI	Patients with PTSD with a new prescription for a SSRI/SNRI

Measures Rationale and Overview

Duration of New SSRI/SNRI Treatment [PTSD-T5]. This measure focuses on whether PTSD patients who received a new prescription for an SSRI/SNRI (no SSRI/SNRI dispensed in the past 90 days) received at least 60 days of medication over an 80-day period. It is adapted from a measure used in the VA evaluation (Farmer et al., 2010), although that measure, unlike this one, required an adequate SSRI/SNRI for all PTSD patients with an NTE. A trial of an SSRI or SNRI should be optimized before shifting to a new treatment strategy. The measure is based on a recommendation in the VA/DoD Clinical Practice Guideline (2010) that medication side effects and response to medication be monitored for a minimum of eight weeks before a clinician proceeds to a new treatment trial for nonresponsive patients. The grade for this timing recommendation is 'C,' which indicates that there is "fair" evidence to conclude that the recommendation "can improve health outcomes" but that the "balance of benefits to harms is too close to justify a general recommendation" (VA and DoD, 2010). Given the low grade of evidence supporting the timing for this measure, it will be important to continue to validate this measure to ensure that the threshold provides a maximized opportunity for an SSRI/SNRI to begin to reduce symptoms while minimizing the length of the time spent on unsuccessful medication trials. Medication treatment in itself is not necessarily indicated by this quality measure because both medication and psychotherapy are appropriate options, but if medications are selected, appropriate management is important.

Follow-up of New Prescription for SSRI/SNRI [PTSD-T6]. This measure assesses whether a follow-up E&M visit occurred within 30 days after the new medication was first dispensed. This is a newly developed measure that will require validation. The 30-day follow-up window is thought to represent an adequate time period for newly prescribed SSRI/SNRI therapy, allowing the provider to make a determination of initial response and evaluate side effects experienced by the patient (VA and DoD, 2010). The follow-up visit provides an opportunity for the provider to titrate dosage, substitute a different SSRI or SNRI, or discontinue pharmacological treatment (due to medication side effects), as well as provide additional information and support for the patient to enhance patient engagement and adherence since one-third of patients will discontinue treatment within a month of receiving the prescription (Simon, 2002). We

Table 4.9
PTSD Measure Scores Related to Medication Management, 2013–2014

Measure	Numerator[a]	Denominator[a]	Measure Score
Percentage of PTSD patients with a newly prescribed SSRI/SNRI with an adequate trial (≥ 60 days) [PTSD-T5]	1,852	2,547	72.7%
Percentage of PTSD patients newly prescribed an SSRI/SNRI with follow-up visit within 30 days [PTSD-T6]	1,132	2,539	44.6%

[a] Based on administrative data; direct and purchased care.

selected the 30-day time period based on clinical judgment because empirical evidence is not available to support a specific time period. It is important for providers to maintain contact with patients to assess side effects and barriers to medication adherence and treatment engagement.

Measure Results

Of those PTSD patients newly treated with an SSRI/SNRI (PTSD-T5), almost 73 percent filled prescriptions for 60 days or more (Table 4.9). Approximately 45 percent of active-component service members in the PTSD cohort who filled a new prescription for SSRI/SNRI had an E&M follow-up visit within the next 30 days (PTSD-T6).

Of those who failed the duration of SSRI/SNRI measure PTSD-T5, 50.2 percent received a 30-day supply, 19.4 percent received 31 to 45 days of medication, and 23 percent received more than 45 days but less than 60 days. The majority of the patients in the denominator (74.6 percent) received less than or equal to a 30-day supply of medication at the first prescription fill. Because these results were based solely on administrative data, it is not possible to know how many of the patients who failed the measure may have discontinued the medication early for justified reasons (e.g., adverse side effects). It is also possible that dispensed medication may have been supplemented with professional samples that would not have been counted in the total days' supply. This measure is limited to evaluating the days' supply dispensed and does not take into account medication that may have been discontinued by the patient after dispensing.

The denominator for the new prescription follow-up measure (PTSD-T6) is smaller than that for the duration of medication treatment measure (PTSD-T5) due to denominator exclusions (see Appendix A for details). The mean time to the E&M visit for patients who passed this measure was 16.9 days (range: 1–30). For those patients who did not receive care specified by this measure, 16 percent had a follow-up E&M visit between 31 and 45 days later and another 10 percent had a follow-up E&M visit between 46 and 60 days later. Of those patients who passed the measure and had a follow-up E&M visit within 30 days of the new prescription, 77 percent saw a mental health provider at the qualifying follow-up visit.

One consideration when interpreting the follow-up visit measure (PTSD-T6) is that phone, email, and other visits that were not coded as an evaluation and management visit did not qualify for the requisite follow-up visit. Another consideration that may have affected measure scores was the frequent provider use of the CPT code 99499 (*unlisted evaluation and management service*) in the administrative data. Because of its undefined nature and general nonacceptance as a basis for cost reimbursement, this code is not an E&M code that satisfies the numerator requirement for this measure. It is possible that a higher proportion of appropriate care may have been given that was not recognized in the measure scores due to the lack of more specific coding used on the part of the provider. We also analyzed the new SSRI/SNRI prescription follow-up measure (PTSD-T6) with the denominator limited to those with at least two

PTSD diagnoses during the measurement period. This resulted in a measure score of 45.6 percent that is only slightly higher than the score of 44.6 percent for the measure as specified.

Comparative Results from Other Sources

Duration of New SSRI/SNRI Treatment [PTSD-T5]. Comparative data for this measure stems from three studies of veterans. Farmer and colleagues (Farmer et al., 2010) found 27.9 percent of veterans with a PTSD NTE were prescribed SSRIs while in VHA care during FY 2007 with an adequate trial (at least 60 days) of this medication. The specifications for that measure differed from the current study in that the VA measure required a SSRI/SNRI trial for every PTSD NTE patient, and those without SSRI/SNRI treatment did not pass the measure. The measure in our study included only PTSD patients (NTE or otherwise) who were newly prescribed an SSRI/SNRI (and did not require an SSRI/SNRI trial). A different study (Shin et al., 2014) reported that 37 percent of veterans with newly diagnosed PTSD who were given a prescription for an SSRI/SNRI received an adequate trial, defined as a minimum 90-day supply. Jain, Greenbaum, and Rosen (2012) found that of veterans newly diagnosed with PTSD and prescribed a first-line SSRI/SNRI, 61 percent received an adequate trial (continuous 90-day supply of the same SSRI/SNRI). The 2012–2013 score for this measure from Phase I of this study was 69.9 percent (Hepner et al., 2016). The 2013–2014 MHS measure score is slightly higher (72.7 percent). While there is still room to improve on this measure, measure scores are similar to that in the other populations studied.

Follow-Up of New Prescription for SSRI/SNRI [PTSD-T6]. Although there are no available comparative data for PTSD patients, the NCQA reported the percentage with follow-up of at least three visits in the 90 days after a new antidepressant prescription fill date for patients with depression to be 18.7 percent, 10.7 percent, and 22.6 percent for commercial, Medicare, and Medicaid plans, respectively, based on 2007 data (National Committee for Quality Assurance, 2008). The 2012–2013 score for this measure was 45.4 percent in our Phase I study (Hepner et al., 2016), which decreased slightly to 44.6 percent in 2013–2014 in this study. Continued implementation of this

Table 4.10
PTSD Treatment Measures: Psychotherapy, 2013–2014

Measure Title	Measure Statement	Numerator	Denominator
Evidence-based psychotherapy [PTSD-T7]	Percentage of PTSD patients who received evidence-based psychotherapy	Patients who received any evidence-based psychotherapy during the measurement period	PTSD patients who received any psychotherapy
Psychotherapy for a new treatment episode [PTSD-T8]	Percentage of PTSD patients with an NTE who received any psychotherapy within four months	Patients who received any psychotherapy within four months following the start of a new treatment episode	PTSD patients with an NTE

quality measure within DoD would allow for comparison of scores across MHS providers and facilities.

Treatment: Psychotherapy

Two treatment measures address the psychotherapy received by PTSD patients and those with a new treatment episode (Table 4.10).

Measures Rationale and Overview

Evidence-based Psychotherapy [PTSD-T7]. The evidence-based psychotherapy measure was adapted from the VHA Mental Health Program Evaluation (Farmer et al., 2010; Watkins et al., 2011) and is based on clinical care recommendations in *VA/ DoD Clinical Practice Guideline: Management of Posttraumatic Stress* (VA and DoD, 2010). The CPG authors identify trauma-focused psychotherapy and stress inoculation therapy (SIT) as evidence-based psychotherapies for PTSD. Selection of these psychotherapy approaches as the first-line behavioral treatments is consistent with other systematic reviews, including a Cochrane review that concluded that trauma-focused cognitive behavioral therapy/exposure therapy (TF-CBT), stress management (a class that includes SIT), and eye movement desensitization and reprocessing (EMDR) are effective in the treatment of PTSD (Bisson and Andrew, 2007). The American Psychiatric Association's *Practice Guideline for the Treatment of Patients with Acute Stress Disorder and Posttraumatic Stress Disorder* (American Psychiatric Association, 2004) includes the recommendation that CBT be considered for acute and chronic PTSD and that other appropriate treatments include TF-CBT variants (e.g., EMDR, imagery rehearsal) and stress inoculation training. An AHRQ report on treatment for PTSD confirms these conclusions (Jonas et al., 2013). While this measure reflects the treatment recommendations of the PTSD CPG, the challenge remains as to how to increase the effectiveness of psychotherapy for patients with PTSD (Steenkamp et al., 2015; Yehuda and Hoge, 2016).

This measure was applied to all PTSD patients identified using administrative data who received any psychotherapy during the measurement period. Information about the therapy received was abstracted from behavioral health provider psychotherapy session notes found in the medical record. To identify whether psychotherapy delivered was consistent with evidence-based treatment (EBT), we required documentation of at least two of three elements of EBT. Specifically, we assessed whether providers (1) addressed the role of thoughts or cognitions, (2) addressed the role of behaviors, or (3) identified what the patient could do before the next session (i.e., homework) (Cooper et al., 2016). Abstractors looked for these elements in the content of provider notes until at least two were found (or looked in all psychotherapy session notes, if fewer than two elements were found).

Psychotherapy for a New Treatment Episode [PTSD-T8]. This measure utilizes administrative data and assesses whether a patient with a diagnosis of PTSD in a new treatment episode had a cohort diagnosis (primary or secondary) psychotherapy visit within four months of the index visit. It was modified from a measure used in the VHA Mental Health Program Evaluation (Farmer et al., 2010; Sorbero et al., 2010; Watkins et al., 2011). This measure is consistent with VA/DoD *Clinical Practice Guidelines for Management of Posttraumatic Stress* (VA and DoD, 2010), which recommends various forms of psychotherapy as a first-line treatment option. This indicator does not capture the type of psychotherapy offered (i.e., evidence-based or not), nor whether the patient may have chosen to decline an offer of psychotherapy or received medication treatment instead. Further, the threshold for success on the measure is met after a single psychotherapy session, which is unlikely to be adequate to achieve a response. **For these reasons, this indicator is considered a descriptive measure.** Psychotherapy for an NTE was satisfied for this measure with the receipt of any individual or group psychotherapy within four months of the NTE.

Measure Results

The denominator for the evidence-based psychotherapy measure (PTSD-T7) was service members in the MRR sample who had received at least one session of psychotherapy (Table 4.11). About 45 percent of those in the denominator received any therapy that appeared to be consistent with evidence-based psychotherapy, based the presence of at least two EBT components documented in the medical record. The measure did not include a requirement of a minimum number of sessions that met these parameters. The score for this measure when applied to all PTSD service members in the MRR sample was 39.8 percent.

Beyond the findings regarding scores on this measure, additional data collected by MRR abstractors and additional analyses can assist in interpreting these findings. Of the patients who received at least two components of EBT, the types of therapy most frequently cited by the provider in session notes were trauma-focused cognitive behavioral therapy (TF-CBT) (32.8 percent), cognitive processing therapy (CPT) (25.8

Table 4.11
PTSD Measure Scores Related to Psychotherapy, 2013–2014

Measure	Numerator	Denominator	Measure Score
Percentage of PTSD patients who received evidence-based psychotherapy for PTSD [PTSD-T7]	159[a]	351[b]	45.3%
Percentage of PTSD patients in an NTE who received any psychotherapy within four months [PTSD-T8]	1,926[c]	2,600[c]	74.1%

[a] Based on medical record data; direct care only.

[b] Based on administrative data; direct care only.

[c] Based on administrative data; direct and purchased care.

percent), prolonged exposure (PE) (14.5 percent), and EMDR (7.6 percent). The medical record abstractors did not evaluate the content of the psychotherapy provided to classify the type, but rather documented the type of therapy as it was designated in the record by the provider. These percentages do not represent all types of therapy received by the sampled patients, but rather the type of EBT first noted in the medical record. For those patients with at least two elements of EBT, the abstractor also counted the number of sessions with the same provider, starting with the first psychotherapy session that met the minimum requirements for EBT. Based on the abstractor's count of same-provider sessions, the average number of sessions was 9.8 (ranging from one to 57), with a median of seven sessions. We also looked at the frequency of the EBT components (i.e., thoughts, behaviors, and homework) that qualified the therapy as being EBT: 88.1 percent of patients with EBT sessions had the role of thoughts documented in their session notes, 64.8 percent had behavior, and 75.5 percent had homework. These frequencies do not represent all of the components used in the EBT sessions, but rather the first two EBT elements found in the medical record psychotherapy notes.

Information about EBT was challenging for the medical record abstractors to collect due to the volume and complexity of mental health provider notes and the variations in documentation style among providers. Among PTSD measures, abstractor interrater reliability was the lowest for this PTSD measure (PABAK, or prevalence and bias adjusted kappa, of 0.43). Also, 28 patients in the PTSD MRR sample had evidence in the medical record documentation that suggested the existence of a shadow record not accessible to the abstractor.

In the population of only PTSD service members in an NTE, and based on administrative data, 74.1 percent of the PTSD NTEs in the denominator received at least one psychotherapy session (in any setting, by any type of provider) in the first four months after the index visit (PTSD-T8). Of the 674 patients who did not receive this care, 8.6 percent first had psychotherapy in four to six months after the start of the new treatment episode, and another 13.5 percent first had psychotherapy more than six months later. With regard to medication treatment as an alternative for patients who did not receive a psychotherapy visit within four months of an NTE, 75 patients received a 60-day supply of an SSRI/SNRI during the four-month measurement period, suggesting that approximately 77 percent of the denominator received either some psychotherapy or an appropriate course of medication. Limiting the denominator for this measure to those with at least two PTSD diagnoses resulted in a measure score of 82.4 percent, somewhat higher than the 74.1 percent reported here.

Comparative Results from Other Sources

Evidence Based Psychotherapy [PTSD-T7]. Limited comparable data are available for this measure. According to medical-record data in a study of veterans, 19.9 percent of veterans in a PTSD cohort who received psychotherapy in FY 2007 received therapy that included at least two elements of CBT (Farmer et al., 2010). The current study found 45.3 percent of PTSD cohort patients who received psychotherapy received at least two core elements, suggesting they received an EBT. While this measure score is higher than that in Farmer et al. (2010), MHS can still work to ensure a higher percentage of patients with PTSD receive evidence-based psychotherapy.

Psychotherapy for New Treatment Episode [PTSD-T8]. Given that studies use a variety of time frames in examining the percentage with psychotherapy received among PTSD patients starting a new treatment episode, it is difficult to directly compare results. Analysis of VHA administrative data showed 43.1 percent of veterans in a PTSD NTE received any psychotherapy within four months (Sorbero et al., 2010), and another study (Shin et al., 2014) reported that of veterans in a PTSD NTE, 45 percent received any PTSD-related psychotherapy within one year. An examination of veterans newly diagnosed with PTSD in another study found that 39 percent received any behavioral counseling within six months (Spoont et al., 2010). Of veterans who received a new PTSD diagnosis in a VA outpatient facility in FY 2004, 36 percent received at least one psychotherapy visit in the 12 months (Cully et al., 2008). A study of psychotherapy utilization over time (FY 2004, 2007, and 2010) among veterans with newly diagnosed PTSD found that 35.3 percent, 32.8 percent, and 34.2 percent, respectively, received at least one psychotherapy session (Mott et al., 2014). Utilization of psychotherapy during calendar year 2005 by privately insured individuals with PTSD was 74.6 percent (Harpaz-Rotem, Libby, and Rosenheck, 2012). The national sample in the Harpaz-Rotem et al. study was nonrepresentative of the general U.S. population; the individuals selected represented 3 percent to 4 percent of the U.S. population with employer-sponsored health care, and the study did not include data from Medicaid, Medicare, or uninsured patients. The score for this measure in Phase I of this study based on 2012–2013 data was 73.3 percent (Hepner et al., 2016), which increased slightly to 74.1 percent based on 2013–2014 data in this report. Despite the shorter follow-up time frame used in our study (i.e., four months) compared with some of the other studies noted here, the MHS measure score is considerably higher than those reported in the other studies.

Table 4.12
PTSD Treatment Measures: Receipt of Care in First Eight Weeks, 2013–2014

Measure Title	Measure Statement	Numerator	Denominator
Receipt of care in first eight weeks [PTSD-T9]	Percentage of PTSD patients in an NTE who received four psychotherapy visits or two evaluation and management visits within the first eight weeks	Patients who received four psychotherapy visits or two evaluation and management visits within eight weeks of an NTE	PTSD patients with an NTE

Treatment: Receipt of Care in First Eight Weeks

The measure noted in Table 4.12 addresses the care received in the first eight weeks by patients with a new treatment episode of PTSD.

Measure Rationale and Overview

This measure uses administrative data to assess whether a patient with a diagnosis of PTSD in a new treatment episode had four cohort diagnosis (primary or secondary) psychotherapy visits or two evaluation and management visits within the first eight weeks after diagnosis. This measure was developed for this project to assess receipt of a minimally appropriate level of care for PTSD patients entering a new treatment episode. The specification of four psychotherapy visits within eight weeks is consistent with a recommendation in the VA/DoD PTSD clinical practice guideline (VA and DoD, 2010) and with technical specifications used in the VA Mental Health Program Evaluation (Horvitz-Lennon et al., 2009); an alternate level of care of two E&M visits for the purpose of medication management is recommended by the VA/DoD practice guidelines (VA and DoD, 2009). Although the exact number of visits selected is not necessarily based on strong empirical data, it is consistent with the care recommended in the CPGs.

Measure Results

Almost 36 percent of active-component service members with a diagnosis of PTSD received four psychotherapy visits or two evaluation and management visits within eight weeks after the start of a new treatment episode (Table 4.13). The denominator for this measure is smaller than that for the psychotherapy for an NTE measure (PTSD-T8) in the prior section due to denominator exclusions (see Appendix A for details). Of those passing the measure, 54.5 percent passed based on the basis of four psychotherapy visits, 27 percent passed with two E&M visits, and 18.5 percent passed based on having both psychotherapy and E&M visits. Similar to the new SSRI/SNRI prescription follow-up measure (PTSD-T6), scores on the receipt of care measure (PTSD-T9) is affected by provider coding practices. Here, too, the frequent use of the CPT code 99499 (*unlisted evaluation and management service*) by providers could have resulted in a lack of inclusion in the measure numerator of otherwise appropriate care

Table 4.13
PTSD Measure Score for Receipt of Care in Eight Weeks, 2013–2014

Measure	Numerator[a]	Denominator[a]	Measure Score
Percentage of PTSD patients with an NTE who received four psychotherapy visits or two E&M visits in the first eight weeks [PTSD-T9]	925	2,608	35.5%

[a] Based on administrative data; direct and purchased care.

in the absence of more specific coding. Limiting the denominator for this measure to those with at least two PTSD diagnoses resulted in a measure score of 39.4 percent compared with 35.5 percent reported here.

Comparative Results from Other Sources

Comparative results for receipt of care in the literature varied according to the length of follow-up, definition of minimally adequate care, and the patient populations studied. In a study of soldiers diagnosed with PTSD within 90 days of return from deployment to Afghanistan, 41 percent received eight or more PTSD-related encounters in the 12 months following diagnosis (Hoge et al., 2014). Among a sample of veterans newly diagnosed with PTSD, 8 percent received at least eight psychotherapy sessions within a 14-week period (Shin et al., 2014). A report by Spoont and colleagues (2010) of veterans who were diagnosed with PTSD in a VA facility between 2004 and 2005 and received behavioral counseling stated that 24 percent received eight counseling visits in the six months after diagnosis. Given the different definitions of minimally adequate care, it is difficult to make direct comparisons between the results of our study and other findings. Another distinction is that none of the comparative studies explicitly included medication management visits in their definitions of minimally adequate care. The measure score for PTSD-T9 from Phase I of this study was 33.6 percent based on 2012–2013 data (Hepner et al., 2016). Although somewhat higher than the Phase I score, the 2013–2014 measure score (35.5 percent) in the current report is still low, indicating room for improvement on ensuring receipt of an adequate

Table 4.14
PTSD Treatment Measures: Symptom Assessment and Response to Treatment, 2013–2014

Measure Title	Measure Statement	Numerator	Denominator
Periodic symptom assessment with PCL [PTSD-T1]	Percentage of PTSD patients with assessment of symptoms with PCL during the four-month measurement period	Patients with a PCL administered at least once during the four-month measurement period	Patients with a PTSD encounter within the four-month measurement period
Response to treatment at six months [PTSD-T10]	Percentage of PTSD patients with response to treatment at six months	Patients with a reduction of five or more points on the PCL within six months	PTSD patients with a PCL score positive for PTSD (PCL score > 43)
Remission at six months [PTSD-T12]	Percentage of PTSD patients in remission at six months	Patients with a PCL score indicative of PTSD remission (PCL score < 28) within six months	PTSD patients with a PCL score positive for PTSD (PCL score > 43)
Improvement in functional status [PTSD-T14]	Percentage of PTSD patients in a new treatment episode with improvement in functional status at six months	Patients with an improvement in functional status from their first visit for PTSD to six months after the first visit	PTSD patients with an NTE with at least two measures of functional status in the first six months

number of psychotherapy or medication management visits following a new PTSD diagnosis.

Treatment: Symptom Assessment and Response to Treatment

The measures in Table 4.14 assess the assessment of PTSD symptoms over time and the patient response to treatment.

Measures Rationale and Overview

Periodic Symptom Assessment with PCL [PTSD-T1]. This measure is based on clinical care recommendations in *VA/DoD Clinical Practice Guideline: Management of Post-traumatic Stress* (VA and DoD, 2010). The guideline recommends "regular follow-up with monitoring and documentation of symptom status" in the treatment of PTSD in both primary care and mental health specialty settings. In discussing the regularity of monitoring, the guideline recommends that patients be assessed at every treatment visit and encourages clinicians to consider a validated measure, such as the PCL. Comprehensive reassessments and evaluations should occur every three months after initiating treatment for PTSD, to monitor changes in clinical status and revise the intervention plan accordingly. The interval of three months is suggested because many controlled trials of first-line therapies for PTSD recommended in this guideline demonstrate clinically significant changes during this time frame VA and DoD, 2010, p. 94).

There is an increasing emphasis on the need to deliver care that is evidence-based and effective. Harding and colleagues (2011) make the case for measurement-based care as the standard for psychiatric practice to align with physical health care. Standardized, repeated measurement of PTSD symptoms allows clinicians to track individual patient response to treatment and adjust care strategies to optimize patient outcomes. It also allows administrators and organizations to monitor the treatment outcomes of larger patient groups. Greenberg, Rosenheck, and Fontana (2003) have shown that standardized assessment of PTSD symptoms is related to PTSD treatment outcomes. Because of the widespread use of the PCL and its recommended use by the MHS (DoD, 2013), it has been incorporated as the standardized tool to be utilized with these symptom monitoring measures.[4] This measure is patterned after the NQF-endorsed measure No. 0712 that assesses for utilization of the PHQ-9 to monitor patients with MDD (National Quality Forum, 2013a). It has been adapted here for patients with PTSD and use of the PCL to monitor patient response to treatment over time. The measure examines the utilization of the PCL for patients with at least one condition-related encounter during four-month intervals within the 12-month mea-

---

[4] The diagnostic criteria for PTSD were updated in the 2013 revision of DSM-5 (American Psychiatric Association, 2013). A revised version of the PCL (PCL-5) reflects these changes (Weathers et al., 2013). It will be important to track the future use of this instrument and update measure-scoring protocols accordingly.

surement period. The measure requires just one use of the PCL per eligible four-month period and is unrelated to any prior PCL score. Data for the numerator for this measure came from symptom questionnaire data collected through the BHDP. At the time of the data collection, use of the BHDP was limited to the Army. The data analyzed for this measure were also limited to those service members who received only direct care to assure that all care relating to the measure numerator and denominators was available for analysis (i.e., providers of qualifying encounters in the denominator for PTSD-T1 had access to the BHDP). At the time of data collection, the BHDP was primarily used in behavioral health settings. Therefore, the specifications for denominator eligibility were limited to those encounters with a behavioral health provider.

Response to Treatment at Six months [PTSD-T10] and Remission at Six Months [PTSD-T12]. The response to treatment measure [PTSD-T10] and remission measure [PTSD-T12] are patterned after the NQF-endorsed measures Nos. 1884 and 0711 that assess for response to treatment and remission in six months for patients with MDD as measured by the PHQ-9 (National Quality Forum, 2013a). We applied the NQF model of use of the PHQ-9 in MDD to the regular use of the PCL to monitor response to treatment for patients with PTSD. The PCL is a validate measure and that can be used to assess ongoing treatment response in patients with PTSD. The measure denominator includes PTSD patients with a PTSD-related encounter with a behavioral health provider and a PCL score of 44 or higher in the first five months of the measurement period. These are new quality measures and there are arguments for various PCL score cut points to define the denominators. The cut point may be lower in a primary care population to improve case identification versus in behavioral health care. A score of 44 was selected for a broader application; it has been shown to have good sensitivity (0.94), specificity (0.86), and strong diagnostic efficiency (0.90) (Blanchard et al., 1996). Response at six months is defined as a five-point reduction in that score, and remission at six months is defined as a score of 27 or lower. Investigators active in PCL refinement recommend that reductions in scale scores of ten to 20 points be considered clinically meaningful change and that reductions of five to ten points be considered reliable changes (Monson et al., 2008). We selected the minimum five-point threshold for this measure for two reasons. First, it is the threshold used to assess initial response to treatment in the RESPECT-Mil protocol for primary care management of PTSD (Oxman et al., 2008). Although this protocol is designed to assess initial response (after six weeks of care), we maintained the threshold here as a *minimum* standard of care. As treatment facilities are able to maximize performance on this achievable aim, administrators may wish to set new goals for treatment success. The recommended threshold for identifying a patient as a probable PTSD case in a specialty mental health clinic is 45 to 50 (National Center for PTSD, 2012). Thresholds to identify PTSD in primary care settings, where the prevalence of PTSD is much lower, are shifted downward to improve identification (under the assumption that a thorough assessment will occur after the screening). The recommended threshold for identifying possible PTSD in these settings is 30 for both civilians and active-duty service members (Blanchard et al., 1996; Bliese et al., 2008; National Center for PTSD, 2012; Oxman et al., 2008). For this measure, we selected a denominator eligibility threshold that increased the likelihood the score was associated with a probable PTSD diagnosis in the denominator. We selected a PCL score of less than 28 as the metric for remission to be consistent with the remission definition in the RESPECT-Mil protocol for treatment of PTSD in primary care (Oxman et al., 2008).[5] Scores for these measures were calculated using symptom questionnaire data from the BHDP (limited to Army only, direct care only, and behavioral health care).

Improvement in Functional Status [PTSD-T14]. This is a new measure based on the recommendation of the Post-Deployment Health Guideline Expert Panel (DoD, Deployment Health Clinical Center and Panel, 2001). General functioning or health-related quality of life (HRQOL) is widely recognized as an important outcome (Moriarty, Zack, and Kobau, 2003). The postdeployment measure on which the change in function measure is based did not specify the instrument to be used to measure change in function. Clinicians and researchers who wish to track patient function over time and in response to treatment have a variety of function measures from which to choose. However, many of these measures are lengthy (e.g., SF-36: McHorney, Ware Jr., and Raczek, 1993) and some of the most popular short measures are associated with licensing fees (e.g., SDS: Sheehan, Harnett-Sheehan, and Raj, 1996; EQ-5D: Rabin and Charro, 2001). The Centers for Disease Control Health-Related Quality of Life "Healthy Days" instrument (CDC HRQOL-4) (Centers for Disease Control and Prevention, 2000) is a good option that balances the need for a validated instrument of functioning with a preference for a brief and no-cost instrument. Although the CDC-HRQOL has been used as a population health surveillance measure, to our knowledge, it has not been implemented as part of a quality measure. This measure assesses for improvement in function based on measurements with a standardized tool within six months of an NTE and is determined from data collected from the medical record. Since no particular tool is required, medical record abstractors were given a list of example tools to search for, including those mentioned above as well as the Brief Resilience Scale (Smith et al., 2008), Global Quality of Life (Hyland and Sodergren, 1996), WHO Disability Assessment Scale (WHODAS) (Garin et al., 2010), Schwartz Outcomes Scale-10 (SOS-10) (Blais et al., 1999), and the Illness Management and Recovery (IMR) Scale (Sklar et al., 2012), but were also instructed to include and document the use of any other standardized tool measuring function.

---

[5]   RESPECT-Mil total scale scores for the PCL (Oxman et al., 2008) are an algebraic transformation from the original Blanchard and colleagues (1996) PCL scoring. To convert RESPECT-Mil PCL thresholds to conventional scale scores, add 17 to the RESPECT-Mil PCL score.

Table 4.15
PTSD Measure Scores Related to Symptom Monitoring and Response to Treatment, 2013–2014

Measure	Numerator	Denominator	Measure Score
Percentage of PTSD patients with symptom assessment with PCL during the four-month measurement period [PTSD-T1]			
Months 1–4	1,187[a]	2,697[b]	44.0%
Months 5–8	810[a]	1,578[b]	51.3%
Months 9–12	832a	1,343[b]	62.0%
Overall	2,829[a]	5,618[b]	50.4%
Percentage of PTSD patients with PCL score > 43 with reduction of PCL score of at least five points at six months [PTSD-T10]	171[a]	916[a,b]	18.7%
Percentage of PTSD patients with PCL score > 43 with a PCL score < 28 at six months [PTSD-T12]	11[a]	916[a,b]	1.2%
Percentage of PTSD patients with an NTE with improvement in function in six months [PTSD-T14]	NR[c]	229[b]	NR

NOTE: NR = not reportable.

[a] Based on symptom questionnaire data; direct care only.

[b] Based on administrative data; direct care only.

[c] Based on medical record data; direct care only.

Measure Results

Utilization of the PCL at least once for patients with a PTSD-related encounter during four-month intervals of the observation period ranged from 44 to 62 percent over the measurement period (Table 4.15). Since each four-month interval is considered separately, a patient may be eligible for one, two, or three intervals. We also computed an aggregate score of minimal utilization for all three of the four-month periods and obtained a score of 50.4 percent. PCL response rates (PTSD-T10) and remission rates (PTSD-T12) were rather low at 18.7 percent and 1.2 percent, respectively. These results include those patients with a triggering score and no follow-up score in the five-to-seven-month interval. The percentage of patients with a triggering score and a follow-up score measured five to seven months later was 41.7 percent. This indicates that 58.3 percent of those in the measure denominator did not have a follow-up PCL in the six-month window (five to seven months after the triggering score). The change in function measure (PTSD-T14) was not reportable due to the lack of regular use by providers in the MRR sample of a standardized tool to measure function. The medical record data revealed that of 229 PTSD patients with NTEs, less than 2 percent had a baseline measurement of function with a standardized tool within 30 days of the NTE. If the MHS cites function as a measureable outcome of interest and recommends the consistent use of a particular standardized tool for this purpose, this measure could be applied in the future. The results reported for response (PTSD-T10) and remission (PTSD-T12) are unadjusted rates and, therefore, should be interpreted with caution. More work would need to be done to develop a risk-adjustment model for these measures.

Comparative Results from Other Sources

Periodic Symptom Assessment with PCL [PTSD-T1]. We identified one previous study that examined rates of periodic PTSD symptom assessment. Farmer and colleagues (2010) found 0.3 percent of veterans with a PTSD NTE in FY 2007 had at least four documented assessments of PTSD symptom severity with a standardized tool within a year. Of all patients in the PTSD cohort in the Farmer study (2010), 4.2 percent had at least one assessment of PTSD symptoms using a standardized instrument during the 12-month study period. Although not directly comparable, reported rates for the use of the PHQ-9 in depression (NQF-endorsed measure on which this measure was patterned) by the Minnesota Community Measurement for the four-month period from October 2012 to January 2013 was 66 percent (National Quality Forum, 2013a). The Minnesota group has been measuring and publishing Minnesota results for measures related to depression and other conditions since 2004 (MN Community Measurement, undated). In our study, PCL utilization rates for the three four-month measurement periods (months 1–4, months 5–8, and months 9–12) were 44.0, 51.3, and 62.0 percent, respectively. These scores indicate an increasing percentage of the PTSD service members with a PTSD-related encounter had at least one PCL per eligible four-month period. Following mandates of PCL use for PTSD assessment in the MHS, measure scores across MHS branches, facilities, and providers would be expected to continue to increase.

Response to Treatment at Six Months [PTSD-T10]. Farmer et al. (2010) attempted to assess reduction in target symptoms among veterans with a PTSD NTE, but because of the limited use of standardized tools to assess symptoms in that study, no veterans met the denominator criteria for this comparative indicator. While not related to PTSD, reported results for response in depression patients using the PHQ-9 in 2013–2014 reported by the Minnesota Community Measurement was 12 to 13 percent (MN Community Measurement, undated). Our study found 18.7 percent of service members in the PTSD cohort with baseline PCL scores greater than 43 had at least a five-point reduction in PCL scores within six months of treatment. This relatively low measures score indicates room for improvement in the response of service members to PTSD treatment.

Remission at Six Months [PTSD-T12]. Our review of the literature found no comparative data for this measure. As an aside, reported results for remission in depression patients using the PHQ-9 in 2013–2014 in Minnesota was 7 to 8 percent (MN Community Measurement, undated). The PTSD remission rate in this study was just 1 percent. Implementation of this quality measure within DoD would allow for comparison between providers, MTFs, and branches across the MHS.

Improvement in Functional Status [PTSD-T14]. The postdeployment measure on which this measure is based did not specify the instrument to be used to measure change in function. The MHS does not currently recommend a single standardized tool for use.

Treatment: Psychiatric Discharge Follow-up

The following measure assesses the outpatient follow-up of patients with PTSD who have been discharged from an inpatient psychiatric hospitalization (Table 4.16).

Measure Rationale and Overview

This measure assesses whether follow-up occurred within specified periods of time after discharge (i.e., seven and 30 days) from a hospitalization with a mental health discharge diagnosis among patients with a diagnosis of PTSD. This is an NQF-endorsed measure that is also part of the NCQA Healthcare Effectiveness Data and Information Set (HEDIS) 2015 measure set (National Committee for Quality Assurance, 2015b), although the HEDIS and NQF measures are not restricted to PTSD patients. The 2010 VA/DoD Clinical Practice Guideline for PTSD (VA and DoD, 2010) refers to the potential use of case management to coordinate and increase continuity of care. Research evidence also supports this measure. Missed appointments and similar disengagement from mental health services may lead to exacerbation of psychiatric symptoms, repeated hospitalizations, first-episode or recurrent homelessness, violence against others, and suicide (Dixon et al., 2009; Fischer et al., 2008; Mitchell and Selmes, 2007; U.S. Government Accountability Office, 2014). The measure score was computed using administrative data. The denominator included inpatient discharges with a primary mental health diagnosis. (For details, see Appendix A.) The requisite follow-up could be an outpatient visit, intensive outpatient encounter, or partial hos-

Table 4.16
PTSD Treatment Measures: Psychiatric Discharge Follow-up, 2013–2014

Measure Title	Measure Statement	Numerator	Denominator
Follow-up after hospitalization for mental illness[a] [PTSD-T15]	Percentage of psychiatric hospital discharges among patients with PTSD with follow-up within • seven days [PTSD-T15a] • 30 days [PTSD-T15b]	Inpatient discharges with an outpatient encounter with a mental health practitioner within • seven days [PTSD-T15a] • 30 days [PTSD-T15b]	PTSD patients discharged from an acute inpatient setting with a primary mental health diagnosis

[a]NQF-endorsed measure.

pitalization. The measure looks for follow-up in the seven and 30 days after discharge. The follow-up contact must be with a behavioral health provider and may occur anytime during the two time windows, including the day of discharge.

Measure Results

Among the PTSD cohort, 87.6 percent and 96.1 percent of active-component service members with a diagnosis of PTSD discharged with a primary mental health diagnosis had a follow-up visit within seven days and 30 days, respectively (Table 4.17).

Of those who passed the seven-day measure (PTSD-T15a), 40.3 percent had their follow-up visit on the day of discharge, and 31.7 percent had the visit one day after discharge. A total of 85.4 percent of patients had their follow-up visit within 72 hours of discharge. Of patients who passed the 30-day measure (PTSD-T15b), 96.6 percent had their first follow-up within 14 days of discharge and 98.6 percent within 21 days. There is some controversy about including in the numerator a follow-up visit that occurred on the same day as hospital discharge. Computing the scores for this measure while requiring a follow-up on post-discharge Day 1 or later resulted in just slightly lower seven-day and 30-day scores: 80.4 percent and 95.4 percent, respectively.

Comparative Results from Other Sources

Follow-Up after Hospitalization for Mental Illness [PTSD-T15a, PTSD-T15b]. Comparative data for this measure come from analyses of both military and civilian populations. An evaluation of VHA mental health services (Sorbero et al., 2010) found that of veterans diagnosed with PTSD who received VA services during FY 2007, 51.3 percent and 82.1 percent received a follow-up outpatient visit within seven and 30 days of acute psychiatric inpatient discharge, respectively. Note that this evaluation considered only the first mental health discharge in the study period, compared with the present study, which included all qualifying discharges. For patients across all mental health diagnoses (not just PTSD) in commercial, Medicaid, and Medicare HMO plans in 2014, the follow-up visit scores are 53.0, 43.9, and 35.3 percent, respectively, within seven days of an MH-related discharge, and 71.0, 63.0, and 54.3 percent, respectively, within

Table 4.17
PTSD Measure Scores Related to Follow-up After Hospitalization for Mental Illness, 2013–2014

Measure	Numerator[a]	Denominator[a]	Measure Score
Percentage of psychiatric hospital discharges among patients with PTSD with follow-up within			
• Seven days [PTSD-T15a]	1,629	1,859	87.6%
• 30 days [PTSD-T15b]	1,786	1,859	96.1%

[a] Based on administrative data; direct and purchased care.

30 days (National Committee for Quality Assurance, 2015b). For those in commercial or Medicare PPO plans in 2014, follow-up visit scores are 49.6 and 34.7 percent, respectively, within seven days of an MH-related discharge, and 69.2 and 56.7 percent, respectively, within 30 days (National Committee for Quality Assurance, 2015b). In a review of MHS care, percentages with follow-up care after discharge from MH-related hospitalizations were 58.5 percent within seven days and 74.8 percent within 30 days for direct care, and 34.4 percent within seven days and 57.4 percent within 30 days for those with purchased care (DoD, 2014c). The scores for this measure from Phase I of this study from 2012–2013 data were 85.7 percent and 95.3 percent (PTSD-15A, PTSD-T15b, respectively) (Hepner et al., 2016). In this study, scores for follow-up care were comparable but slightly higher within seven days (87.6 percent) and 30 days (96.1 percent) of mental health–related discharge for service members with a diagnosis of PTSD. It is important to note that MHS recently issued a memo that stressed the importance of follow-up care within 72 hours of discharge and suggested avoiding discharge on weekends and federal holidays to support this effort (Department of the Army Headquarters, 2014a), which may have played an important role in stimulating efforts to enhance follow-up. Further study may help uncover additional mechanisms MHS implemented to achieve such high levels of performance in this arena.

Quality of Care for PTSD over Time and by Service Branch, TRICARE Region, and Service Member Characteristics, Based on Administrative Data

Examining patterns over time, five of the six PTSD measure scores based on administrative data increased slightly between 2012–2013 and 2013–2014. The largest increase was nearly 3 percentage points in having a new minimum 60-day SSRI/SNRI filled prescription (PTSD-T5). However, the percentage with follow-up visit within 30 days of a new SSRI/SNRI prescription for PTSD (PTSD-T6) decreased slightly over this time period.

In our prior work, we examined variation in 2012–2013 quality measure scores by service branch, TRICARE region, and service member characteristics, including age, gender, race/ethnicity, pay grade, and deployment history for the administrative data–based quality measures (Hepner et al., 2016). Several large and statistically significant differences in quality of care were observed across branches of service and TRICARE region. While the variations in care were not consistent across measures, the results still raised concerns about whether care is consistent and equitable across the variables we examined in the MHS.

We updated results for the administrative data–based quality measures using 2013–2014 data to examine whether these variations in care remained. The quality of PTSD care varied substantially by service branch and TRICARE region. Percentages

Table 4.18
Summary of Service and Member Characteristics with Statistically Significant Differences in 2013–2014 Quality Measure Scores for PTSD

PTSD Measure	Service Branch	Region	Age	Race/ Ethnicity	Gender*	Pay Grade	Deployment History
New SSRI/SNRI for ≥ 60 days (T5)		X		X			
Visit in 30 days after new SSRI/SNRI (T6)		X					
Psychotherapy within 4 months of NTE (T8)						X	X
Care within 8 weeks of NTE (T9)							X
Visit in 7 days after MH discharge (T15a)	X		X				
Visit in 30 days after MH discharge (T15b)	X		X				

X = One or more statistically significant differences ($P < 0.05$) among subgroups defined by this characteristic.

* The measure scores for two PTSD measures, T8 (psychotherapy within four months of NTE) and T15a (visit in 7 days after MH discharge) differed significantly between males and females before the P-values were adjusted for multiple comparisons, but differences were not significant after the adjustment.

Table 4.19
Summary of Statistically Significant Differences in 2013–2014 Quality Measure Scores, by Service and Member Characteristics for PTSD

PTSD Measure	Significant Results
New SSRI/SNRI for ≥ 60 days (T5)	Region: West > South Race/Ethnicity: White, non-Hispanic/Other-Unknown > Black, non-Hispanic
Visit in 30 days after new SSRI/SNRI (T6)	Region: Overseas > South
Psychotherapy within 4 months of NTE (T8)	Pay Grade: E1–E4/E5–E9 > O4–O6 Deployment History: Not deployed > Deployed
Care within 8 weeks of NTE (T9)	Deployment History: Not deployed > Deployed
Visit in 7 days after MH discharge (T15a)	Age: 25–34 > 18–24 Branch: Army/Air Force > Marine Corps/Navy
Visit in 30 days after MH discharge (T15b)	Age: 25–34 > 18–24 Branch: Army/Air Force > Marine Corps/Navy

NOTE: Comparisons between subgroups listed in this table showed a statistically significant difference at $P < 0.05$.

with follow-up visits within seven days of mental health discharge (PTSD-T15a) differed across service branches by as much as 16 percent for the PTSD cohort. Percentages with visits within 30 days of a new SSRI/SNRI prescription (PTSD-T6) for the PTSD cohort showed variation across TRICARE regions by up to 12 percent. We also observed significant disparities in quality of care by service member characteristics. For the PTSD cohort, percentages with psychotherapy within four months of beginning an NTE (PTSD-T8) differed by as much as 15 percent across pay grades. The PTSD cohort also saw variations in measure scores by race/ethnicity. Percentages with adequate filled prescriptions of SSRI/SNRIs (PTSD-T5) differed across racial categories by up to 13 percent for the PTSD cohort. The large observed differences in PTSD quality measure scores by service branch, TRICARE region, and service member characteristics suggest that similar variation in the quality of PTSD care was observed in 2013–2014 as in 2012–2013.

In Table 4.18, we highlight the characteristics for which measure scores showed statistically significant variation for the PTSD measures in 2013–2014. For the subgroups that exhibit statistically significant differences, additional information on the direction of the differences for each measure is detailed in Table 4.19. A set of charts illustrating the variation in PTSD measure scores by these characteristics is available in Appendix D.

Summary

In the following list, we highlight key findings from this chapter assessing care for PTSD.

PTSD Measures: Key Findings

- **Assessment** of active-component service members beginning an NTE of PTSD for **comorbid depression, suicidal ideation, and recent substance use** was high in this sample (93–96 percent) and equaled or outperformed comparative veteran populations.
- **Assessment of baseline symptom severity** of PTSD for a new treatment episode with the PCL was not as frequent (47 percent, as represented by the medical record), though current efforts are under way within the MHS to increase the regular use of the PCL to monitor PTSD patient symptoms.
- **Standardized tools** were used in less than half of the assessments for depression, suicide risk, and recent substance use and almost never used for assessment of function.
- Appropriate **minimal care for patients with suicidal ideation** was less than optimal (54 percent), primarily due to a lack of documentation regarding address-

ing access to lethal means. A Safety Plan Worksheet has recently been added to the clinical guideline for assessment and management of suicide risk which may improve this performance in the future.

- Adequate **duration of new SSRI/SNRI treatment** was 73 percent, similar to or better than other comparative scores. However, a smaller percentage (45 percent) had an **evaluation and management visit** within 30 days of the newly prescribed SSRI/SNRI.

- Most PTSD patients with an NTE receive **psychotherapy** in the first four months after diagnosis. But among PTSD patients who received psychotherapy, just 45 percent received any therapy that contained at least two elements consistent with evidence-based therapy.

- A low proportion (36 percent) of PTSD patients beginning an NTE received an adequate amount of **care (either psychotherapy or evaluation and management visits) in the eight weeks following the start of an NTE.**

- Rates of **minimal use of the PCL** over the 12-month measurement period showed continuous increase over the three four-month intervals (44, 51, and 62 percent), although re-measurement rates at five to seven months for those with a PCL score > 43 was 42 percent. Rates of **response and remission** based on PCL scores were low (19 percent and 1 percent, respectively).

- **Follow-up after hospitalization for a mental health diagnosis** in patients with PTSD continued to be very high compared with other health care systems, with 88 percent seen within seven days and 96 percent within 30 days.

- Comparing **results over time**, five of the six PTSD measure scores based on administrative data increased slightly between 2012–2013 and 2013–2014. The largest increase was nearly 3 percentage points in having a new minimum 60-day SSRI/SNRI filled prescription. However, the percentage with a follow-up visit within 30 days of a new SSRI/SNRI prescription for PTSD decreased slightly over this time period.

- Comparing **results by service characteristics**, measure scores by service branch differed up to 16 percent for follow-up after mental health discharge. Measure scores by TRICARE region differed up to 12 percent for visits after a new SSRI/SNRI prescription.

- Comparing **results by member characteristics**, measure scores by pay grade differed up to 15 percent for psychotherapy within four months of beginning an NTE. Measure scores by race/ethnicity differed up to 13 percent for adequate filled prescriptions of SSRI/SNRIs.

CHAPTER FIVE

Quality of Care for Depression

Depression Quality Measure Scores, 2013–2014

In this chapter, we present the results of analyses **focused on the outpatient care provided** to active-component service members for depression using the quality measures based on administrative data, MRR, and symptom questionnaire data collected through the BHDP. These measures, based on CPGs, are outlined in Chapters One and Two, and technical specifications are detailed extensively in Appendix B.[1] **The administrative data measures represent outpatient care provided in both direct care and purchased care settings. We analyzed outpatient medical record data for a smaller sample of active-component service members who received only direct care provided by MTFs. The measures based on symptom questionnaire data represent active-component service members in the Army who received direct care only and visits to behavioral health specialty care.** Table 5.1 shows the characteristics of the service members contained in each data type. Many characteristics of the three groups are similar. However, those in the MRR sample and the group with symptom questionnaires were limited to service members who received direct care only. The symptom questionnaire group was also limited to those in the Army. The depression MRR sample differed from the other two because it was stratified to include a larger proportion of service members beginning an NTE (i.e., 59 percent in the MRR sample versus 25 percent in the cohort and 29 percent in the symptom questionnaire sample). Utilization of care for the depression MRR sample was also less than the other two, perhaps a reflection of the higher proportion of NTEs. The MRR and symptom questionnaire samples both had lower utilization than the cohort, perhaps reflecting the limitation of those samples to service members with direct care only. The overlap among the three groups is shown in Figure 5.1. The care provided to each service member with a depression diagnosis should be consistent with the depression guidelines as assessed by the quality measures, even among those who also have a diagnosis of PTSD.

---

[1] Appendixes for this report are available online: http://www.rand.org/pubs/research_reports/RR1542.html.

Table 5.1
Characteristics of Service Members with Depression in the Cohort, MRR Sample, and with Symptom Questionnaire Data Used to Calculate Quality Measure Scores

Characteristic	Cohort % (N)	MRR Sample % (N)	Symptom Questionnaire % (N)
Total	100 (30,496)	100 (400)	100 (5,195)
Gender			
Female	33.6 (10,239)	32.5 (130)	27.1 (1,406)
Race/ethnicity			
American Indian/Alaskan native	1.4 (436)	1.5 (6)	0.9 (48)
Asian/Pacific Islander	4.4 (1,327)	6.5 (26)	5.4 (278)
Black, non-Hispanic	19.4 (5,929)	20.8 (83)	23.9 (1,239)
White, non-Hispanic	60.3 (18,385)	58.0 (232)	57.0 (2,960)
Hispanic	11.7 (3,579)	10.8 (43)	12.1 (626)
Other	2.8 (840)	2.5 (10)	0.8 (44)
Age			
18–24	23.2 (7,069)	31.3 (125)	22.2 (1,152)
25–34	44.0 (13,424)	40.5 (162)	44.4 (2,309)
35–44	27.6 (8,428)	26.3 (105)	28.2 (1,466)
45 and over	5.2 (1,575)	2.0 (8)	5.2 (268)
Service			
Army	55.7 (16,980)	52.0 (208)	100 (5,195)
Air Force	19.1 (5,833)	16.3 (65)	NA
Marine Corps	8.5 (2,601)	12.5 (50)	NA
Navy	14.0 (4,280)	19.3 (77)	NA
Coast Guard	2.6 (802)	NA	NA
Region			
North	24.9 (7,604)	21.8 (87)	16.1 (835)
South	29.7 (9.044)	23.8 (95)	29.5 (1,530)
West	32.6 (9,931)	35.5 (142)	31.5 (1,636)
Overseas	11.1 (3,398)	19.0 (76)	21.3 (1,109)
Unknown	1.7 (519)	NA	1.6 (85)

Table 5.1—Continued

Characteristic	Cohort % (N)	MRR Sample % (N)	Symptom Questionnaire % (N)
Never deployed[a]	32.0 (9,745)	31.0 (124)	22.9 (1,190)
Have a new treatment episode (NTE)	25.0 (7,637)	58.5 (234)	28.5 (1,481)
Direct care only	43.1 (13,138)	100 (400)	100 (5,195)
Received any acute inpatient care	21.9 (6,667)	13.3 (53)	12.3 (641)
Received any inpatient care with a primary mental health discharge diagnosis	12.6 (3,829)	5.0 (20)	5.9 (306)
Median outpatient encounters for any diagnosis (for those with at least one)	31	21.5	26
Median outpatient encounters with a primary mental health diagnosis (for those with at least one)	11	7	10

[a] Based on data from September 2001 through March 2015

Figure 5.1
Three Sources for Depression Measure Denominators

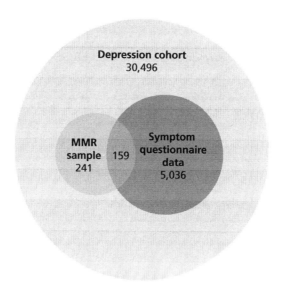

In the following sections, we present the results of our evaluation of care for depression. Each quality measure focuses on the subset of patients who met the eligibility requirements as specified in the measure denominator. Measure denominators have specifications that not all patients will meet, such as starting a new medication, having a particular type of health care encounter, or starting a new treatment episode. As a result, 46 percent of the depression cohort were included in at least one administrative data quality measure denominator, 95 percent of the MRR sample were included in at least one medical record–based measure, and 87 percent of the symptom questionnaire group were included in at least one measure using symptom questionnaire data. First, we present measure scores for the MHS. When available, we provide prior data from other health care systems, or prior data from the MHS, on the same or related quality measures to provide context to interpret results and inform whether the quality measure should be a target for quality improvement. We then evaluate variations by patient characteristics, service branch, and TRICARE region for quality measures based on administrative data.

Assessment: Symptom Severity and Comorbidity

The four measures in Table 5.2 focus on the assessments of symptom severity and comorbidity for patients with a new treatment episode of depression.

Measures Rationale and Overview

These measures were adapted from the VHA Mental Health Program Evaluation (Farmer et al., 2010; Watkins et al., 2011). Measure Depression-A3 is also an NQF-endorsed measure for patients with newly diagnosed MDD. Information about symp-

Table 5.2
Depression Assessment Measures: Symptom Severity and Comorbidity, 2013–2014

Measure Title	Measure Statement	Numerator	Denominator
Baseline symptom assessment with the PHQ-9 [Depression-A1]	Percentage of depression patients with an NTE with assessment of symptoms with the PHQ-9 within 30 days	Patients with an assessment of depression symptoms within 30 days	Depression patients with an NTE
Assessment for mania/hypomania [Depression-A2]	Percentage of depression patients with an NTE assessed for manic or hypomanic behaviors within 30 days	Patients assessed for symptoms or behaviors associated with mania or hypomania within 30 days	Depression patients with an NTE
Assessment for suicide risk[a] [Depression-A3]	Percentage of depression patients with an NTE assessed for suicide risk at the same visit	Patients assessed for current suicide risk during the NTE visit	Depression patients with an NTE
Assessment for recent substance use [Depression-A4]	Percentage of depression patients with an NTE assessed for substance use within 30 days	Patients assessed for recent substance use, including type, quantity, and frequency, within 30 days	Depression patients with an NTE

[a] NQF-endorsed measure.

tom severity and comorbidity is necessary to guide the development of an appropriate treatment plan.

Baseline Symptom Assessment with the PHQ-9 [Depression-A1]. The VA/DoD CPG for major depression (VA and DoD, 2009) states that the PHQ-9 ought to be used as part of an initial assessment for any patient with a positive depression screen or for whom depression is suspected and used as an adjunct assessment tool even when a full diagnostic interview is conducted. Harding and colleagues (2011) make the case for measurement-based care as the standard for psychiatric practice to align with physical health care. The PHQ-9 is a nine-item self-report measure of symptoms of depression that is simple to administer and score (Kroenke, Spitzer, and Williams, 2001). The PHQ-9 is recommended by the MHS for monitoring depression symptoms (DoD, 2014e). Consistent with the NQF-endorsed measure specifications for monitoring symptoms of MDD over time (No. 0712) (National Quality Forum, 2015b), we specify the use of the PHQ-9 to establish an objective, baseline score and means for monitoring the patient's response to treatment over time.

Assessments for Mania/Hypomania [Depression-A2] and Recent Substance Use [Depression-A4]. The VA/DoD CPG also recommends assessing the newly diagnosed depression patient for a range of psychiatric comorbidities, including bipolar disorder and substance use, to plan treatment accordingly. The assessment measures for screening for behaviors of mania and hypomania (Depression-A2) and recent substance use (Depression-A4) required the use of either a standardized tool or an informal assessment within 30 days of diagnosis. The substance use screen was satisfied with an assessment for either alcohol or drug use. If an informal assessment was used for drug use (Depression-A4), it needed to include an assessment of type and frequency of use, and for alcohol use, it needed to include amount and frequency of use. The 30-day time frame includes assessments in the 30 days before through the 30 days after to include assessments that may have been performed just prior to or shortly after the diagnosis of the condition.

Assessment for Suicide Risk [Depression-A3]. The VA/DoD CPG also recommends assessing the patient for safety and risk to self and others. This measure is based on NQF-endorsed measure No. 0104, which requires screening for SI in newly diagnosed patients of MDD (National Quality Forum, 2013a). While the NQF measure targets MDD, we have also applied this measure to the broader population of patients with an NTE of depression (including MDD). As mentioned earlier, the DoD has increased attention on preventing suicide among service members. In 2008, the age-adjusted suicide rate in active-component service members exceeded that in civilians, 20.2 compared with 19.2, respectively (VA and DoD 2013). In calendar year 2014 among active-component service members in all services, the suicide rate was 19.9 per 100,000 (DoD 2016). The 2014 suicide rate varied by branch of service, with Army having the highest rate (23.8 per 100,000) followed by Air Force (18.5 per 100,000), Marine Corps (17.9 per 100,000), and Navy (16.3 per 100,000). The assessment for suicide risk (Depression-A3) needed to have occurred at the same visit as the NTE to pass the measure. This measure allows for the use of a standardized tool or informal assessment but is required to be done at the same visit that started the NTE. If the assessment for suicidal ideation was positive, the measure requires an assessment for presence or absence of a plan and access to means unless the patient was hospitalized.

Measure Results

All numerators for the four assessment measures are based on medical record review data (Table 5.3). Approximately 37 percent of depression patients were assessed with the PHQ-9 within 30 days of beginning an NTE (Depression-A1). Assessment for evidence of mania or hypomania (Depression-A2) was completed for only a quarter of service members (25.6 percent). Of the 60 patients screened for mania/hypomania (Depression-A2), all were screened informally without the use of a standardized tool. Assessments for suicide risk (Depression-A3) and recent substance use (Depression-A4) were performed more frequently, at 87.6 percent and 90.2 percent, respectively. For

Table 5.3
Depression Measure Scores Related to Assessment of Symptom Severity and Comorbidity, 2013–2014

Measure	Numerator[a]	Denominator[b]	Measure Score (%)
Percentage of depression patients with an NTE with assessment of symptoms with the PHQ-9[c] [Depression-A1]	87	234	37.2
Percentage of depression patients with an NTE assessed for mania/hypomania [Depression-A2]	60	234	25.6
Percentage of depression patients with an NTE assessed for suicide risk [Depression-A3]			
MDD NTEs (NQF diagnostic codes)[d]	39	45	86.7
Depression NTEs (cohort diagnostic codes)	205	234	87.6
Percentage of depression patients with an NTE assessed for recent substance use [Depression-A4]	211	234	90.2

[a] Based on medical record data; direct care only.

[b] Based on administrative data; direct care only.

[c] Unlike other measures utilizing the PHQ-9 (T1, T10, and 12), which were scored using BHDP data, measure Depression-A1 numerator was scored using data from the medical record, since abstractors were collecting data for the other three assessments (Depression A2, A3, and A4). While BHDP PHQ-9 scores are intended to be entered into the medical record, this may not happen in every instance. Therefore, a limitation of the data used for this measure is that a score entered within 30 days of the NTE into the BHDP would have been missed if not also entered into the medical record. Prior to curtailing data collection, we looked at a small sample of patients and compared scores from the BHDP data to scores collected from the medical record. At that time, neither source appeared to be superior in that while some scores were identical in the two sources, others were missing from either source with similar frequency.

[d] NQF-endorsed measure.

the assessment of suicide risk measure, we provide the measure score for the patients meeting the NQF specifications for the denominator, as well as the score for the larger group of NTEs with depression (MDD or other depression cohort diagnosis). The two scores were very similar (86.7 percent and 87.6 percent, respectively).

Assessment for suicide risk (Depression-A3) was most often completed as an informal assessment, rather than using a standardized tool (either of which was acceptable). Of the 205 patients (87.6 percent) assessed for suicide risk on the date of NTE, a standardized tool was used with 42 patients (20.5 percent). This was usually the single suicide item from the PHQ-9. Of the 29 patients who did not meet the criteria for assessment for suicide risk, 14 did not have any screen for suicidal ideation. The remaining 15 had a positive screen, but did not have the required documentation of an assessment of the patient's access to lethal means.

When screening for recent substance use (Depression-A4), providers screened 83.3 percent of patients for recent alcohol use and 60.7 percent of patients for recent drug use. While the percentage screened for recent alcohol use is similar to that for PTSD-A4 (80 percent), the percentage with screening for recent drug use (60.7 percent) is lower than for the PTSD sample (83.4 percent). Providers most often used informal screens (76.4 percent for alcohol and 100 percent for drug use), rather than a standardized measure (e.g., the AUDIT-C). When a standardized tool was used to screen for alcohol use, the tool of choice was the AUDIT-C (73.9 percent), followed by the AUDIT (26.1 percent).

Comparative Results from Other Sources

Assessment of Depression with the PHQ-9 [Depression-A1] and Assessment for Mania/Hypomania [Depression-A2]. Our review of the literature did not identify any similar results for comparison for these measures. However, implementation of these quality measures within DoD would allow for comparison of measure scores across MHS providers and sites.

Assessment for Suicide Risk (Depression-A3). Suicide assessment rates among patients with depression varied widely across studies. Analysis of data in the 2010 CMS Physician Quality Reporting Initiative (PQRI) shows 96.6 percent of patients with a new diagnosis of MDD received a suicide risk assessment at that visit (National Quality Forum, 2014a). The percentage with suicide risk assessment was 81.8 percent for veterans who received services from the VHA in FY 2007 for at least one of the following diagnoses: schizophrenia, bipolar I disorder, PTSD, major depression, or substance use disorders (Farmer et al., 2010). That metric represented the percentage of veterans in the study who had at least one screen for SI in the medical record during the 12-month measurement period. A secondary data analysis found 24 percent of primary care patients who either (1) tested positive for MDD or dysthymia on the Composite International Diagnostic Interview (CIDI) or (2) tested negative but reported at least five of nine depression criteria were assessed for suicidal ideation by a primary care provider (Hepner et al., 2007). In our study, the percentage of service members with depression who were assessed for suicide (86.7 percent for MDD, 87.6 percent for MDD or depression) is higher than in most other studies.

Assessment for Recent Substance Use (Depression-A4). Comparative data for this measure are only available for care provided by the VHA. Of veterans who received VHA primary care and screened positive for depression (i.e., scored 10 or higher on the PHQ-9), 64.9 percent were assessed for current drug or alcohol use (Dobscha et al., 2003). An evaluation of VHA care found 72 percent of veterans in the MDD cohort who received care during FY 2007 received an alcohol or drug use assessment within 30 days of an MDD NTE (Farmer et al., 2010). Our study found a relatively high percentage of active-component service members with depression received an assessment for recent substance use (90.2 percent), suggesting that this assessment is well integrated into routine care for service members diagnosed with depression.

Treatment: Follow-up for Suicidal Ideation

The following measure focuses on the assessment and treatment of service members who presented with suicidal ideation (Table 5.4).

Measure Rationale and Overview

A similar follow-up measure was used in the VHA Mental Health Program Evaluation (Farmer et al., 2010; Watkins et al., 2011). That measure has been significantly modified here based on the newer *VA/DoD Clinical Practice Guideline for Assessment and Management of Patients at Risk for Suicide* (VA and DoD, 2013). This CPG specifies that the recommended course of treatment for SI be tied to a clinical judgment of whether the acute risk for suicide is low, intermediate, or high. That acute risk status judgment (low, intermediate, high) is then mapped onto several possible clinical responses. When acute risk status is low, the provider can choose to consult with a behavioral health provider or address the safety issues and treat the presenting problems without such a consult. When acute risk status is intermediate, the minimum recommendations are to limit access to lethal means, conduct a complete behavioral evaluation (or refer to a behavioral health provider to do so), and determine an appro-

Table 5.4
Depression Treatment Measures: Follow-up for Suicidal Ideation, 2013–2014

Measure Title	Measure Statement	Numerator	Denominator
Appropriate follow-up for endorsed suicidal ideation [Depression-T3]	Percentage of patient contacts of depression patients with SI with appropriate follow-up (Depression-T3)	Patients with appropriate follow-up on the same day that SI was documented	Depression patient visit where positive suicidal ideation was documented

priate referral. When acute risk status is high, the guidelines recommend maintenance of direct observational control of the patient and transfer to an emergency care setting for hospitalization.

We had planned to limit application of the suicidal ideation follow-up measure (Depression-T3) to a smaller subset of patients whose providers had assessed and documented the patient's level of suicide risk as low, intermediate, or high. The level of risk, based on other assessments of comorbid risk and supportive factors, determined the minimum interventions required for appropriate care for this measure. However, only 15 patients (28.3 percent) with SI had a documented high/intermediate/low risk level. This may well reflect the very recent release of the suicide risk CPG at the time of data collection. Enough time may not have elapsed after publication of the CPG for the diffusion of its content and general implementation throughout the MTFs. Therefore, we opted to apply a single minimal level of required follow-up care for all 53 patients with SI that included (for patients not hospitalized) three required elements: (1) an assessment for plan and access to lethal means, (2) a referral or appointment for follow-up, and (3) a discussion of limitation of access to lethal means or documentation that the access assessment was negative. These requirements follow the recommendations in the CPG's decisionmaking Algorithm A for low-risk patients (suicide CPG, VA and DoD, 2013). The care assessed was limited to that related to the first episode of suicidal ideation noted in the record during the measurement period.[2] Appropriate care needed to have been provided on the same day that the SI was documented.

Measure Results

During medical record review, abstractors identified 53 depression patients with at least one occurrence of suicidal ideation. For 44 of these patients (83.0 percent), a behavioral health provider documented the positive SI. Among the 53 patients with positive SI, 16 (30.2 percent) had documentation of all three elements of the recommended care on the same day when SI was noted. For all 37 patients where recommended care was not documented, there was a failure to address lethal means (i.e., no documented discus-

Table 5.5
Depression Measure Score for Follow-up of Suicidal Ideation, 2013–2014

Measure	Numerator[a]	Denominator[a]	Measure Score
Percentage of patient contacts of depression patients with SI with appropriate follow-up (Depression-T3)]	16	53	30.2%

[a] Based on medical record data; direct care only.

---

[2] The time period for identifying SI was initially the entire 12 months of the measurement period, but this was later reduced during the medical record abstraction to the first six months due to time constraints. See Chapter Two, Methods.

sion of limiting access to lethal means and no assessment or a positive assessment for access to means) (Table 5.5).

We also summarized the types and frequencies of suicide-related assessments performed at the visit where the positive SI was documented (Table 5.6). These assessments represent indicators of risk and contributing factors highlighted in the CPG that could assist the provider in determining the overall level of the patient's suicide risk, and thereby guide the delivery of appropriate care (VA and DoD, 2013). More than half of the patients (64.2 percent) were assessed for the persistence of the SI (i.e., constant, intermittent, or present in the past two weeks) and 83 percent for the level of the patient's intent (i.e., presence or absence of intention to act on the SI). A large percentage (92.5 percent) was assessed for the presence of a suicide plan. Fewer patients (35.8 percent) were assessed for access to means to carry out a suicide. The corresponding percentage of assessing for lethal means in the sample of PTSD patients with SI was 70.8 percent. The overall level of suicide risk was classified as high, intermediate, or low for just 28.3 percent of patients. Few patients (less than 6 percent) had documented information about the presence or absence of recent suicidal behavior. Percentage of patients with documented assessments for recent and prior suicide attempts was 64.2 percent and 75.5 percent, respectively. Providers documented assessments for recent and prior substance use for 75.5 and 47.2 percent of patients, respectively.

We also summarized the interventions taken by providers in treating the 53 patients with SI at the time of the visit (Table 5.7). A behavioral health provider had seen most patients (86.8 percent), and 18.9 percent were hospitalized. For those not

Table 5.6
Risk Factor Assessments of Service Members with Depression Performed on the Same Day the Suicidal Ideation Was Documented

Assessed for Presence or Absence of:[a]	All Patients with Positive SI (n = 53) % (N)
SI persistence	64.2 (34)
Intent	83.0 (44)
Plan	92.5 (49)
Access to means	35.8 (19)
Suicide risk level assigned as high, intermediate, or low	28.3 (15)
Recent suicidal behavior	NR
Recent suicide attempt	64.2 (34)
History of prior attempt	75.5 (40)
Recent substance use	75.5 (40)
History of prior substance use	47.2 (25)

[a] Based on medical record data; direct care only. NR = not reported (cells with fewer than five).

Table 5.7
Interventions for Service Members with Depression on the Same Day the Suicidal Ideation Was Documented

Intervention	All Patients with Positive SI (n = 53) % (N)
Hospitalized[a]	18.9 (10)
Assessed by behavioral health provider[a]	86.8 (46)
For those not hospitalized:	(n = 43)
Lethal means discussion or documented negative assessment for access to means[a]	23.3 (10)
Referral to behavioral health or with the same provider[a]	97.7 (42)
Next visit with any provider occurred within:[b]	
1 week	76.7 (33)
2 or more weeks	23.3 (10)
Next visit with a mental health provider occurred within:[b]	
1 week	65.1 (28)
2 or more weeks	32.6 (14)

[a] Based on medical record data; direct care only.

[b] Based on administrative data; direct care only.

hospitalized, less than a quarter (23.3 percent) had documentation of counseling about limiting access to lethal means or a negative assessment for access to means. The corresponding percentage of PTSD patients in the MRR sample with SI was 44.4 percent. Almost all (97.7 percent) patients who were not hospitalized after assessment were given a referral to a behavioral health provider and/or were instructed to follow up with the same provider. Based on administrative data, 65.1 percent of the 43 patients not hospitalized subsequently had a visit within one week with a mental health provider and 76.7 percent with any provider.

Comparative Results from Other Sources

Appropriate Follow-up for Endorsed Suicidal Ideation [Depression-T3]. We found limited comparative data for this measure. Of veterans who received VHA care in FY 2007 for at least one of five psychological disorders (schizophrenia, bipolar I disorder, PTSD, major depression, or substance use disorder), 96.4 percent received appropriate follow-up for suicidal ideation on the same date the SI was documented (Farmer et al., 2010). The abstractors determined appropriateness of the follow-up provided, which included assessment (for intent, plan, and means) and interventions applied (in the absence of hospitalization) such as discussion of safety, provision of a list of appropriate resources, and appointment for follow-up. Discretion was left to the abstractor to determine whether the follow-up was appropriate based on documented data about the patient in the medical record. In our study, abstractors collected data elements about the assessments and follow-up, and the appropriateness of follow-up was determined in analysis according to the requirements noted earlier.

As we noted with the results for PTSD-T3 in Chapter Four, the results we present for follow-up of depression patients with positive SI are based on a relatively small sample of patients and reflect care during a time when the CPG for suicide risk management had only recently been published (June 2013). The 18-month window for this study included a cohort selection window from January through June 2013 and observation of care in the subsequent 12 months that could have continued as long as through June of 2014. Therefore, there may have been only limited uptake of the CPG during the time we observed care. Given the importance of this focus of care, we have made a concerted effort to carefully collect data related to the CPG, particularly those cited as important for determining the level of suicide risk and appropriate action (Table 1, p. 48 of the CPG; DoD/VA, 2013). We also guided our abstraction content based on input from DoD and VA experts. These data are intended to provide an opportunity for the MHS to begin to identify areas of strength and areas that might be the focus of future improvement efforts. Since this study was initiated, a Safety Plan Worksheet (VA, 2014) was added to the 2013 CPG for suicide risk management, and it incorporates limitation of access to lethal means. Generalized use of this tool could facilitate improved performance of this measure.

Treatment: Medication Management

The two measures that address medication management consider the duration of a newly prescribed antidepressant for patients with depression and a follow-up evaluation in the 30 days following dispensing of the medication (Table 5.8).

Measures Rationale and Overview

Duration of Antidepressant Treatment [Depression-T5]. This measure is NQF-endorsed and has been part of the HEDIS Quality Measurement set. This indicator is consistent with recommendations in the VA/DoD Clinical Practice Guideline for Management of Major Depressive Disorder (2009). The guideline strongly recommends antidepressant medications as a first-line treatment option for patients with MDD (see also Fournier et al., 2010; Moncrieff, Wessely, and Hardy, 2004). The VA/DoD Clinical Practice Guideline is consistent with the civilian treatment guideline issued by the American Psychiatric Association (Glenberg et al., 2010). The APA also recommends antidepressants as a treatment option for depression, and for patients who respond to antidepressants, that treatment be continued for four to nine months to reduce the risk

Table 5.8
Depression Treatment Measures: Pharmacologic Therapy Management, 2013–2014

Measure Title	Measure Statement	Numerator	Denominator
Duration of antidepressant treatment [a] [Depression-T5]	Percentage of depression patients with a newly prescribed antidepressant medication for • 12 weeks (acute phase) [Depression T5a] • six months (continuation phase) [Depression T5b]	Antidepressant treatment for • at least 84 days (12 weeks) of continuous treatment with antidepressant • at least 180 days (six months) of continuous treatment with antidepressant	Depression patients with a new prescription for an antidepressant
Follow-up of new prescription for antidepressant [Depression-T6]	Percentage of depression patients newly prescribed an antidepressant with follow-up visit within 30 days	Depression patients with a follow-up visit within 30 days of the new prescription for an antidepressant	Depression patients with a new prescription for an antidepressant

[a] NQF-endorsed measure.

of relapse. Similarly, the Institute for Clinical Systems Improvement guideline recommends antidepressants for patients with depression, indicating the time to remission can take as long as three months, and the medication should be continued for six to 12 months for patients who respond to antidepressants (Trangle et al., 2012). This measure was operationalized using administrative data and followed the technical specifications of the NQF-endorsed measure (No. 0105) (National Quality Forum, 2014b).

Follow-up of New Prescription for Antidepressant [Depression-T6]. This measure was recently developed (Hepner et al., 2015) and will require validation. The 30-day follow-up window is thought to represent an opportunity for the provider to make a determination of initial response and evaluate side effects experienced by the patient (VA and DoD, 2010). The follow-up visit provides an opportunity to titrate dosage, substitute a different SSRI or SNRI, or discontinue pharmacological treatment (due to medication side effects), as well as to provide additional information and support for the patient to enhance patient engagement and adherence since one-third of patients will discontinue treatment within a month of receiving the prescription (Simon, 2002). We selected the 30-day time period based on clinical judgment, because empirical evidence is not available to support a specific time period. It is important for providers to maintain contact with patients to assess side effects and barriers to medication adherence and treatment engagement. Thus, this measure assessed whether a follow-up E&M visit occurred within 30 days after the medication was first dispensed. It was operationalized using administrative data.

Measure Results

Of those depression patients newly treated with an antidepressant, 65 percent filled prescriptions for at least 12 weeks (Depression-T5a) and 46 percent filled prescriptions for at least six months (Depression-T5b). Approximately 41 percent of active-component service members in the depression cohort who filled a new prescription for an antidepressant had an E&M follow-up visit within the next 30 days (Depression-T6) (Table 5.9).

Of those who failed the 12-week version of the antidepressant duration measure (Depression-T5a), 32.2 percent received a 30-day supply, 8.9 percent received 31 to 45 days of medication, and 46.6 percent had a 60-day supply or more but less than the minimum of 84 days' supply. Of those who failed the six-month version of the measure (Depression-T5b), 13 percent had a 90-day supply, and 10 percent had a 120-day supply. Another 27.5 percent had more than a 120-day supply but less than the minimum 180 days. The majority of the patients in the denominator (71.9 percent) received less than or equal to a 30-day supply of medication at the first prescription fill. Because these results were based solely on administrative data, it is not possible to know how many of the patients who failed the measure may have discontinued the medication early for justified reasons (e.g., adverse side effects). It is also possible that dispensed medication may have been supplemented with professional samples that would not have been counted in the total days' supply. This measure is limited to evaluating the supply of medication dispensed and does not take into account medication dispensed but not taken by the patient.

The denominator for the follow-up visit measure (Depression-T6) is smaller than for the antidepressant duration measure (Depression-T5) due to denominator exclusions (see Technical Specifications for details). The mean time to the E&M visit for patients who passed this measure was 16.8 days (range: 1–30). For those patients who failed the quality measure, 14 percent had a follow-up E&M visit between 31 and 45 days, and another 8 percent had a follow-up E&M visit between 46 and 60 days later. Of those patients who passed the measure and had a follow-up E&M visit within 30

Table 5.9
Depression Measure Scores Related to Pharmacologic Therapy, 2013–2014

Measure	Numerator[a]	Denominator[a]	Measure Score (%)
Depression patients who receive a newly prescribed antidepressant for[b]			
• 12 weeks [Depression-T5a]	5,430	8,314	65.3
• six months [Depression-T5b]	3,784	8,222	46.0
Percentage of depression patients newly prescribed an antidepressant with follow-up visit within 30 days [Depression-T6]	3,396	8,216	41.3

[a] Based on administrative data; direct and purchased care.

[b] NQF-endorsed measure.

days of the new prescription, 60 percent saw a mental health provider at the qualifying follow-up visit. We also computed the measure score for a denominator limited to those with at least two depression diagnoses during the observation year, which resulted in a measure score of 44 percent, only slightly higher than what we report.

One consideration when interpreting the follow-up visit measure (Depression-T6) is that phone, email, and other visits not coded as an evaluation and management visit did not qualify for the requisite follow-up visit. Another consideration that may have affected measure scores was the frequent provider use of the CPT code 99499, (*unlisted evaluation and management service)* in the administrative data. Because of its undefined nature and general nonacceptance as a basis for cost reimbursement, this code is not an E&M code that satisfies the numerator requirement for this measure. It is possible that a higher proportion of appropriate care may have been given that was not recognized in the measure scores due to the lack of more specific coding used on the part of the provider.

Comparative Results from Other Sources

Duration of Antidepressant Treatment [Depression-T5a, DepressionT5b]. A recent report to the Secretary of Defense listed MHS measure scores as 68.5 and 46.1 percent for acute and continuation phase antidepressant management, respectively (DoD, 2014c). An earlier evaluation of VHA services reported 48.4 percent and 31.2 percent of veterans with a new treatment episode of MDD filled prescriptions for antidepressants for a 12-week supply (acute phase) and six-month supply (continuation phase), respectively (Sorbero et al., 2010). Among a sample of veterans with a new depressive episode in 2007, 62.6 percent received at least 84 days of an antidepressant (acute phase), and 36.9 percent received at least 180 days (continuation phase) (Jordan et al., 2014). Based on aggregate HEDIS data, effective acute phase treatment measure scores in 2014 were 66.2, 52.3, and 68.5 percent for eligible patients across commercial, Medicaid, and Medicare HMO plans, respectively (National Committee for Quality Assurance, 2015a). Effective acute phase treatment rates in 2014 were 66.0 and 71.6 percent, respectively, for commercial and Medicare PPO plans (National Committee for Quality Assurance, 2015a). Measure scores for continuation phase treatment for commercial, Medicaid, and Medicare HMOs in 2014 were 49.9, 37.1, and 54.7 percent, respectively; for commercial and Medicare PPOs, the scores were 50.6 and 58.4 percent, respectively (National Committee for Quality Assurance, 2015a). The MHS scores for this measure from Phase I of this study for 2012–2013 were 64.4 percent and 44.0 percent (Depression-T5a, Depression-T5b, respectively) (Hepner et al. 2016), which increased somewhat to 65.3 percent and 46.0 percent, respectively, in the current study. While these measure scores are similar to several of those presented as comparative data, MHS has an opportunity to ensure a higher percentage of service members with depression receive an antidepressant prescription for an adequate amount of time.

Follow-up of New Prescription for Antidepressant [Depression-T6]. A study (Chen et al., 2010) analyzed 2000–2002 data on patients 18 years or older who were diagnosed with MDD and initiated treatment with second-generation antidepressants. The authors found that 31 percent of these patients received at least three follow-up visits during the first 90 days after the index antidepressant prescription, and at least one of the follow-up visits was with a provider with prescribing privileges. In Phase I of this study, the MHS score for this measure for 2012–2013 was 42.1 percent (Hepner et al. 2016), while the current study finds the score has decreased slightly to 41.3 percent based on 2013–2014 data. Although the results indicate room to improve, we do not know the ideal expected performance on this measure.

Treatment: Psychotherapy

Two treatment measures address the nature of psychotherapy received by all depression patients and those with a new treatment episode (Table 5.10).

Measures Rationale and Overview

Evidence-Based Psychotherapy [Depression-T7]. This measure comes from the VHA Mental Health Program Evaluation (Farmer et al., 2010; Watkins, Pincus, Paddock, et al., 2011). This measure is consistent with the recommendations of the VA/DoD Clinical Practice Guideline for Management of Major Depressive Disorder (2009). This guideline identifies CBT, interpersonal psychotherapy (IPT), and problem solving therapy (PST) as evidence-based psychotherapies for MDD with the strongest, most extensive evidence base. Practice guidelines from the American Psychiatric Association acknowledge this evidence and include CBT as an appropriate first-line treatment for MDD (Glenberg et al., 2010). The denominator for this measure was service members in the MRR sample who had received at least one session of psychotherapy. Information about the therapy received was abstracted from behavioral health provider psycho-

Table 5.10
Depression Treatment Measures: Psychotherapy, 2013–2014

Measure Title	Measure Statement	Numerator	Denominator
Evidence-based psychotherapy [Depression-T7]	Percentage of depression patients who received evidence-based psychotherapy	Patients who received any evidence-based psychotherapy	Depression patients who received any psychotherapy
Psychotherapy for a new treatment episode [Depression-T8]	Percentage of depression patients with an NTE who received any psychotherapy within four months	Patients who received any psychotherapy within four months of the NTE	Depression patients with an NTE

therapy session notes found in the medical record. We focused on identifying whether the psychotherapy provided was consistent with CBT, as this is the recommended psychotherapy for depression that providers report using most frequently (Hepner et al., 2009). To identify whether the psychotherapy delivered was consistent with CBT for depression, we required documentation of at least two of three core elements of CBT. Specifically, we assessed whether providers (1) addressed the role of thoughts or cognitions, (2) addressed the role of behaviors, or (3) identified what the patient could do before the next session to (i.e., homework). Abstractors looked for these elements documented in provider notes until at least two were found (or looked in all psychotherapy session notes, if fewer than two elements were found). If the psychotherapy did not meet the threshold for CBT, abstractors would then assess whether the provider mentioned the therapy as being either IPT or PST. Abstractors did not evaluate or code elements of these psychotherapy approaches to determine whether the documentation indicated consistency with IPT or PST.

Psychotherapy for a New Treatment Episode [Depression-T8]. This measure uses administrative data to assess whether a patient with a diagnosis of depression had a cohort diagnosis (primary or secondary) visit for psychotherapy (in any setting and with any provider) within four months of beginning a new treatment episode. It was modified from a measure used in the VA Mental Health Program Evaluation (Farmer et al., 2010; Sorbero et al., 2010; Watkins et al., 2011). This measure is consistent with VA/DoD Clinical Practice Guidelines for Management of Major Depressive Disorder (2009) and Posttraumatic Stress (2010), which recommend psychotherapy as a first-line treatment option. This indicator does not capture the type of psychotherapy offered (i.e., evidence-based or not), nor whether the patient may have chosen to decline an offer of psychotherapy or received medication treatment instead. Further, the threshold for success on the measure is met after a single psychotherapy session (of any modality, such as individual or group therapy), which is unlikely to be adequate to achieve a response. **For these reasons, this indicator is considered a descriptive measure.**

Table 5.11
Depression Measure Scores Related to Psychotherapy, 2013–2014

Measure	Numerator	Denominator	Measure Score (%)
Percentage of depression patients who received evidence-based psychotherapy for depression [Depression-T7]	103[a]	345[b]	29.9
Percentage of depression patients in an NTE who received any psychotherapy within four months [Depression-T8]	4,064[c]	7,225[c]	56.2

[a] Based on medical record data; direct care only.

[b] Based on administrative data; direct care only.

[c] Based on administrative data; direct and purchased care.

Measure Results

About 30 percent of depression service members in the MRR sample who received any psychotherapy received any therapy that appeared consistent with CBT, based on medical record review and at least two EBT components (Depression-T7) (Table 5.11). The measure did not include a requirement of a minimum number of total sessions that met these parameters. For all patients with depression in the MRR sample the score was 25.8 percent. About 56 percent of the depression NTEs in the cohort received at least one psychotherapy session in the first four months.

We also looked at additional information to help interpret these findings. Of the service members whose therapy appeared consistent with CBT, the frequency of the CBT components (first two components noted in the record) was 79.6 percent for thoughts, 50.5 percent for behavior, and 81.6 percent for homework. Among the 242 patients who did not pass the threshold for CBT, 4.5 percent and 1.2 percent had documentation they were using IPT or PST, respectively, in the medical record psychotherapy session notes (but these were not included in the numerator because core elements of these therapies were not coded). For those patients with at least two elements of CBT, the abstractor also counted the number of sessions with the same provider, starting with the first psychotherapy session that met the minimum requirements for CBT. The average number of sessions was 7.3 (range: 1–55) with a median of 4.5 sessions. We also computed this measure with a denominator limited to those patients with at least two depression diagnoses during the 12-month observation period, which resulted in a measure score of 29.3 percent, almost the same as the score in Table 5.11 (29.9 percent).

Information about CBT was challenging for the medical record abstractors to collect due to the volume and complexity of mental health provider notes and the variations in documentation style among providers. Among depression measures, abstractor interrater reliability was the lowest for this depression measure, with a PABAK of 0.61. The number of CBT sessions counted by the abstractors may be somewhat underestimated because three patients receiving CBT transferred from the MTF during treatment to continue care with a different provider. In those cases, abstractors stopped counting the CBT sessions and did not evaluate whether or not CBT continued with the next provider. Also, 30 patients in the MRR depression sample had evidence in the medical record documentation that suggested the existence of a shadow record not accessible to the abstractor.

Of the 3,161 patients who did not meet criteria for any psychotherapy for an NTE (Depression-T8), 5.1 percent first had psychotherapy within four to six months after the start of the new treatment episode, and another 9.1 percent first had psychotherapy more than six months later. Medication and psychotherapy are both appropriate treatment options, and a patient might have switched off one and onto another or had one added to augment response. Of those who did not meet the measure criteria, 790 patients received a 12-week supply of an antidepressant during the four-month measurement period, suggesting that approximately 67.2 percent of the denominator received either some psychotherapy or an appropriate course of medication. When this measure was computed limiting the denominator to those with at least two depression diagnoses, the measure score was 68.7 percent, somewhat higher than the score in Table 5.11 (56.2 percent).

Comparative Results from Other Sources

Evidence-Based Psychotherapy [Depression-T7]. Receipt of evidence-based psychotherapy for depression varied across populations. According to a review of VHA mental health care (Farmer et al. 2010), 30.9 percent of veterans in the MDD cohort with at least one psychotherapy visit in FY 2007 received therapy that included at least two elements of CBT. Among a sample of primary care patients across the United States with depression being treated with psychotherapy, 55 percent received psychotherapy with at least one element of CBT (Hepner et al., 2007). The MHS score for this measure (29.9 percent) was similar to the earlier VHA result but still has room for improvement.

Psychotherapy for a New Treatment Episode [Depression-T8]. Given the variability in time frames used to measure psychotherapy receipt after an NTE for depression, it is difficult to directly compare our results to findings of other studies. Among veterans in the MDD cohort with an NTE in FY 2007, 40.3 percent received any psychotherapy within four months (Sorbero et al. 2010). Another study of veterans newly diagnosed with depression in FY 2004 found 18 percent of veterans received at least one visit that involved individual therapy, group therapy, or a combination of the two within 90 days of diagnosis (Burnett-Zeigler et al., 2012). An analysis of veterans diagnosed with new onset depression in FY 2004 reported 21 percent of patients received at least one psychotherapy session in the year following index date (Cully et al., 2008). Of veterans newly diagnosed with MDD in FY 2010 at a VHA outpatient clinic, 26.2 percent received at least one psychotherapy visit during the 12-month follow-up period (Mott et al., 2014). Among a sample of privately insured individuals with an MDD diagnosis in 2005, 62.4 percent received at least one outpatient individual, group, or family psychotherapy session during the calendar year (Harpaz-Rotem, Libby, and Rosenheck, 2012). The 2012–2013 measure score for psychotherapy for a new treatment episode of depression was 52.0 percent (Hepner et al., 2016). The 2013–2014 measure score increased over 4 percentage points to 56.2 percent in the current report. While there is room for improvement, these scores are higher than those of other studies, particularly considering the shortened time frame we used to assess performance.

Treatment: Receipt of Care in First Eight Weeks

One measure addressed the care received in the eight weeks after beginning an NTE for depression (Table 5.12).

Table 5.12
Depression Treatment Measures: Receipt of Care in First Eight Weeks, 2013–2014

Measure Title	Measure Statement	Numerator	Denominator
Receipt of care in first eight weeks [Depression-T9]	Percentage of depression patients with an NTE who received four psychotherapy visits or two evaluation and management visits within the first eight weeks	Patients who received four psychotherapy visits or two evaluation and management visits within eight weeks of the NTE	Depression patients with an NTE

Measure Rationale and Overview

This measure uses administrative data to assess whether a patient with a diagnosis of depression in a new treatment episode had four cohort diagnosis (primary or secondary) psychotherapy visits or two E&M visits (for medication management) within the first eight weeks following the start of an NTE for depression. This measure was developed for this project to assess receipt of a minimally appropriate level of care for depression patients entering a new treatment episode (Hepner et al., 2015). The VA/DoD Clinical Practice Guidelines for MDD do not state explicitly the minimum or optimal number of visits during the initial treatment period (VA and DoD, 2009). However, the measure is consistent with a key element of the MDD guideline that states that "patients require frequent visits early in treatment to assess response to intervention, suicidal ideation, side effects, and psychosocial support systems" (VA and DoD, 2009). The specification of four psychotherapy visits within eight weeks is consistent with technical specifications used in the VA Mental Health Program Evaluation (Horvitz-Lennon et al., 2009). An alternate level of care of two evaluation and management visits for the purpose of medication management is recommended by the VA/DoD practice guidelines (VA and DoD, 2009).

Measure Results

About 25 percent of active-component service members with a diagnosis of depression received four psychotherapy visits or two evaluation and management visits within eight weeks following the start of a new treatment episode (Table 5.13).

The denominator for this measure is smaller than that for the "any psychotherapy" for an NTE measure (Depression-T8) due to denominator exclusions (see Appen-

Table 5.13
Depression Measure Scores Related to Receipt of Care in the First Eight Weeks, 2013–2014

Measure	Numerator[a]	Denominator[a]	Measure Score
Percentage of depression patients in an NTE who received four psychotherapy visits or two E&M visits in the first eight weeks [Depression-T9]	1,757	7,009	25.1%

[a] Based on administrative data; direct and purchased care.

dix B for details). Of those passing the measure, 34.9 percent passed based on the basis of at least four psychotherapy visits, 44.9 percent passed with two E&M visits, and 20.1 percent passed based on having both psychotherapy and E&M visits. Similar to follow-up for antidepressant prescription (Depression-T6), scores on this measure (Depression-T9) are affected by provider coding practices. Here, too, the frequent use by providers of other, nonqualifying procedure codes (e.g., CPT code 99499, *unlisted evaluation and management service*) could have caused otherwise appropriate care to go unrecognized in the numerator requirement for this measure. With a denominator limited to having at least two depression diagnoses, the measure score was 30.6 percent, slightly higher than the score in Table 5.13 (25.1 percent).

Comparative Results from Other Sources

Results are not directly comparable to those of our study, given the difference in population, time frame, and specifications of care. These comparative data come from an analysis of depression care received after hospitalization. Pfeiffer and colleagues (2011) found among a sample of veterans discharged from a psychiatric inpatient stay with an MDD diagnosis, 12.9 percent received at least eight psychotherapy visits within 90 days of discharge. The MHS 2012–2013 score for this measure from Phase I of this study was 23.8 percent (Hepner et al., 2016). While the measure score improved slightly in 2013–2014 (25.1 percent in the current report), the relatively low percentage of service members who passed this measure suggests MHS should work to ensure more active-component service members with depression receive adequate care within eight weeks of diagnosis.

Treatment: Symptom Assessment and Response to Treatment

The following measures focus on assessment of depression symptoms over time and patient response to treatment (Table 5.14).

Measures Rationale and Overview

Periodic symptom assessment with PHQ-9 [Depression-T1]. This measure assessed the utilization of the PHQ-9 in eligible patients with MDD or dysthymia. It is an NQF-endorsed measure (No. 0712) (National Quality Forum, 2015b). The measure is based on clinical care recommendations consistent with the VA/DoD Clinical Practice Guideline for MDD (VA and DoD, 2009), which recommends that the PHQ-9 be used to monitor treatment response following the initiation of treatment and after each change in treatment. Guidelines issued by the Institute for Clinical Systems Improvement also recommend the PHQ-9 as the preferred tool to monitor depression in the primary care setting (Trangle et al., 2012). There is an increasing emphasis on the need to deliver care that is evidence-based and effective. Harding and colleagues (2011)

Table 5.14
Depression Treatment Measures: Symptom Assessment and Response to Treatment, 2013–2014

Measure Title	Measure Statement	Numerator	Denominator
Periodic symptom assessment with PHQ-9 [Depression-T1]	Percentage of depression patients with assessment of symptoms with PHQ-9 during the four-month assessment period	Patients with a PHQ-9 administered at least once during the four-month measurement period	Patients with a depression encounter within the four-month measurement period
Response to treatment at six months [Depression-T10]	Percentage of depression patients with response to treatment at six months	Patients with a six-month PHQ-9 score reduced by at least 50% from the initial PHQ-9 score	Depression patients with a PHQ-9 score positive for depression (> 9)
Remission at six months [Depression-T12]	Percentage of depression patients in remission at six months	Patients with a six-month PHQ-9 score < 5	Depression patients with a PHQ-9 score positive for depression (> 9)
Improvement in functional status [Depression-T14]	Percentage of depression patients with an NTE with improvement in functional status at six months	Patients with an improvement in functional status from their first visit for depression at six months	Depression patients with an NTE who have at least two measures of functional status during the first six months

make the case for measurement-based care as the standard for psychiatric practice to align with physical health care. Standardized, repeated measurement of depression symptoms allows clinicians to track individual patient response to treatment and allows administrators and organizations to monitor the treatment outcomes of larger patient groups. The measure examines the utilization of the PHQ-9 for patients with at least one condition-related encounter during four-month intervals within the measurement period. The measure requires just one use of the PHQ-9 per eligible four-month period and is unrelated to any prior PHQ-9 score. Data for the numerator for this measure came from symptom questionnaire data collected through the BHDP. At the time of data collection, use of the BHDP was limited to the Army. The data analyzed for this measure were also limited to those service members who received only direct care to ensure that all care relating to the measure numerator and denominator was available for analysis (i.e., providers of qualifying encounters in the denominator had access to the BHDP). At the time of data collection, the BHDP was primarily used in behavioral health settings. Therefore, the specifications for denominator eligibility were limited to those encounters with a behavioral health provider.

Response to Treatment at Six Months [Depression-T10] and Remission at Six Months [Depression-T12]. This pair of measures examines response to treatment in six months and remission in six months in patients with a PHQ-9 score of 10 or higher (National Quality Forum, 2013a); they have received NQF endorsement as No. 1884 and No. 0711, respectively. Response is defined as a 50-percent reduction in PHQ-9 score and remission as a PHQ-9 score of less than 5. The measure is consistent with the VA/DoD Clinical Practice Guideline for MDD (VA and DoD, 2009), which recommends that the PHQ-9 be used to monitor treatment response following the initiation of treatment and after each change in treatment. The guideline authors score the strength of this recommendation a "B," which corresponds to the judgment that "at least fair evidence was found that the intervention improves health outcomes and concludes that benefits outweigh harms" (VA and DoD, 2009). Guidelines issued by the Institute for Clinical Systems Improvement also recommend the PHQ-9 as the preferred tool to monitor depression in the primary care setting (Trangle et al., 2012).

Improvement in Functional Status [Depression-T14]. This is a new measure based on the recommendation of the Post-Deployment Health Guideline Expert Panel DoD, Deployment Health Clinical Center and Panel, 2001). General functioning or health-related quality of life (HRQOL) is widely recognized as an important outcome (Moriarty, Zack, and Kobau, 2003). The postdeployment measure on which this measure is based did not specify the instrument to be used to measure change in function. Clinicians and researchers who wish to track patient function over time and in response to treatment have a variety of function measures from which to choose. However, many of these measures are lengthy (e.g., SF-36: McHorney, Ware Jr., and Raczek, 1993) and some of the most popular short measures are associated with licensing fees (e.g., SDS: Sheehan, Harnett-Sheehan, and Raj, 1996; EQ-5D: Rabin and Charro, 2001). The Centers for Disease Control Health-Related Quality of Life "Healthy Days" instrument (CDC HRQOL-4) (Centers for Disease Control and Prevention, 2000) balances the need for a validated instrument of functioning with a preference for a brief and no-cost instrument. Although the CDC-HRQOL has been used as a population health surveillance measure, to our knowledge, it has not been implemented as part of a quality measure. This measure assesses for an improvement in function based on measurement with a standardized tool within six months of an NTE. Since no particular tool is required, medical record abstractors were given a list of example tools to search for, including those mentioned above as well as the Brief Resilience Scale (Smith et al., 2008), Global Quality of Life (Hyland and Sodergren, 1996), WHO Disability Assessment Scale (WHODAS) (Garin et al., 2010), Schwartz Outcomes Scale-10 (SOS-10) (Blais et al., 1999) and the Illness Management and Recovery (IMR) Scale (Sklar et al., 2012), but were instructed to include any other standardized tool measuring functional status.

Measure Results

Results for the symptom monitoring and response to treatment measures are shown in Table 5.15. Use of the PHQ-9 for patients with a depression-related encounter during the four-month intervals of the observation period ranged from 33.5 percent to 51.3 percent in the third interval (Depression-T1). Since each four-month interval is considered separately, a patient may be eligible for one, two, or three intervals. We also

Table 5.15
Depression Measure Scores Related to Symptom Monitoring and Response to Treatment, 2013–2014

Measure	Numerator	Denominator	Measure Score (%)
Percentage of depression patients with symptom assessment with PHQ-9 during the four-month measurement period [a] [Depression-T1]			
Months 1–4	781[b]	2,329 [c]	33.5
Months 5–8	524[b]	1,298 [c]	40.4
Months 9–12	593[b]	1,157 [c]	51.3
Overall	1,898[b]	4,784 [c]	39.7
Percentage of depression patients with PHQ-9 score > 9 with 50% reduction of PHQ-9 score at six months[a] [Depression-T10]	55[b]	770[b,c]	7.1
Percentage of depression patients with PHQ-9 score > 9 with a PHQ-9 score < 5 at six months[a] [Depression-T12]	27[b]	770[b,c]	3.5
Percentage of depression patients with an NTE with improvement in function in six months [Depression-T14]	NR[d]	234[c]	NR

[a] NQF-endorsed measure.

[b] Based on symptom questionnaire data; direct care only.

[c] Based on administrative data; direct care only.

[d] Based on medical record data; direct care only.

computed an aggregate rate of minimal utilization over all three of the four-month periods and obtained a rate of 39.7 percent. The percentage of patients with a triggering score and a follow-up score measured five to seven months later was 37.7 percent. This indicates that 62.3 percent of those in the measure denominator did not have a follow-up PHQ-9 in the six-month window. For those service members with a PHQ-9 score of greater than 9 in the first five months of the observation period, response to treatment (Depression-T10) and remission (Depression-T12) rates were 7.1 percent and 3.5 percent, respectively. These results include those patients with a triggering score and no follow-up in the five-to-seven-month interval. Findings for change in function (Depression-T14) were not reportable due to the lack of regular use by providers in the MRR sample of a standardized tool to measure function. The medical record data revealed that of 234 depression patients with NTEs, less than 2 percent had a baseline measurement of function with a standardized tool within 30 days of the NTE. If the MHS cites function as a measureable outcome of interest and recommends the consistent use of a particular standardized tool for this purpose, this measure could be applied in the future.

Results for the periodic symptom assessment (Depression-T1), response to treatment (Depression-T10), and remission (Depression-T12) measures are based on symptom questionnaire data collected through the BHDP. At the time of the data collection, use of the BHDP was limited to the Army. The data analyzed for these measures were also limited to those service members who received only direct care to assure that all care required for the measures' implementation would be available. The results reported for response to treatment (Depression-T10) and remission (Depression-T12) are unadjusted rates and, therefore, should be interpreted with caution. More work is needed to develop a risk adjustment model for these measures.

Comparative Results from Other Sources

Periodic Symptom Assessment with PHQ-9 [Depression-T1]. According to Minnesota Community Measurement NQF documentation, 65.6 percent of patients with depression or dysthymia seen in a sample of Minnesota clinics were assessed with the PHQ-9 between October 1, 2012, and January 31, 2013. We found the percentage of Army soldiers with depression who were periodically assessed with the PHQ-9 during the specified four-month periods (1–4 months, 5–8 months, and 9–12 months) increased from 33.5 percent to 40.4 percent to 51.3 percent. Because of the differences in the MN and the Army populations, these results are not directly comparable. Although these rates could be improved, they indicate PHQ-9 utilization is increasing over time within the Army.

Response to Treatment at Six Months [Depression-T10]. Available comparable data for this measure come from Minnesota Community Measurement. Risk adjustment is recommended if using this measure to compare performance across groups (e.g., clinics). The risk adjustment model used by Minnesota relies on variables that are not clearly applicable to the MHS population (e.g., health plan, distance from care source). Further, results from Minnesota data are not reported for key service member characteristics; thus, it is difficult to draw any direct comparisons. Of patients in Minnesota with an MDD or dysthymia diagnosis in 2010–2011 who were seen in primary or behavioral health care settings and had an initial PHQ-9 score greater than 9, 10.2 percent had a 50-percent reduction or higher in PHQ-9 score in the six months after treatment. Data from the 2013 and 2014 Minnesota Healthcare Quality Reports shows the state average for response to depression treatment at six months to be 11.7 and 12.8 percent (MN Community Measurement, 2013; MN Community Measurement, 2014). The Army score for this measure is 7.1 percent, with 37.7 percent of the eligible sample with a triggering PHQ-9 score who had a follow-up score in the following five to seven months. The follow-up scores noted in the 2014 Minnesota Health Care Quality Report for 2013 and 2014 were 28 and 31 percent (MN Community Measurement, 2014).

Remission at Six Months [Depression-T12]. As with the response measure (T10), there is comparative data for this measure from Minnesota state-level health care reports, and the same cautions apply about comparing their rates to the MHS unadjusted rates (Garrison et al., 2016). According to the 2013 and 2014 Minnesota Community Measurement Quality Health Care Reports, the statewide average rate for depression remission at six months (PHQ-9 score < 5) was 6.9 and 7.7 percent (MN Community Measurement, 2013; MN Community Measurement, 2014). Our study found the Army score for this measure to be 3.5 percent. Again, note that 37.7 percent of the eligible sample had a triggering PHQ-9 score as well as a follow-up score in the following five to seven months.

Improvement in Functional Status [Depression-T14]. The postdeployment measure on which the change in function measure (Depression-T14) is based did not specify the instrument to be used to measure change in function, and the MHS does not currently recommend a single standardized tool for use.

Treatment: Psychiatric Discharge Follow-up

The following measure assesses the outpatient follow-up of patients with depression who have been discharged from an inpatient psychiatric hospitalization (Table 5.16).

Measure Rationale and Overview

This measure assesses whether follow-up occurred within specified periods of time after discharge (i.e., seven and 30 days) for a hospitalization with a mental health discharge diagnosis among patients with a diagnosis of depression. This is an NQF-endorsed measure that is also part of the NCQA Healthcare Effectiveness Data and Information Set (HEDIS) 2015 measure set (National Committee for Quality Assurance, 2015b), although the HEDIS measure is not restricted to patients with a diagnosis of depression. Research evidence also supports this measure. Missed appointments and similar disengagement from mental health services may lead to exacerbation of psychiatric symptoms, repeated hospitalizations, first-episode or recurrent homelessness, violence against others, and suicide (Dixon et al., 2009; Fischer et al., 2008; Mitchell and Selmes, 2007; U.S. Government Accountability Office, 2014). This measure has face validity, and it is the standard of care to provide patients with adequate follow-up after an inpatient psychiatric stay. Furthermore, this measure is widely used by national

Table 5.16
Depression Treatment Measures: Psychiatric Discharge Follow-up, 2013–2014

Measure Title	Measure Statement	Numerator	Denominator
Follow-up after hospitalization for mental illness[a] [Depression-T15]	Percentage of psychiatric hospital discharges among patients with depression with follow-up within • seven days [Depression-T15a] • 30 days [Depression-T15b]	Inpatient discharges followed with an outpatient visit with a mental health practitioner within • seven days [Depression-T15a] • 30 days [Depression-T15b]	Depression patients discharged from an acute inpatient setting with primary mental health diagnosis

[a] NQF-endorsed measure.

reporting programs, as indicated by its inclusion in HEDIS. The measure score was computed using administrative data. The denominator included patients discharged with a primary mental health diagnosis. (For details, see Appendix B.) The requisite follow-up could be an outpatient visit, intensive outpatient encounter, or partial hospitalization. The measure looks for follow-up in the seven and 30 days after discharge. The follow-up contact must be with a behavioral health provider and may occur anytime during the two time windows, including the day of discharge.

Measure Results

As shown in Table 5.17, among the depression cohort, 87.1 percent and 95.2 percent of active-component service members with a diagnosis of depression discharged with a primary mental health diagnosis had follow-up within seven days and 30 days, respectively, based on our analysis of administrative data (Depression-T15a, Depression-T15b).

Of those who passed the measure at the seven-day level (Depression-T15a), 43.6 percent had their follow-up visit on the day of discharge, and 29.0 percent had the visit one day after discharge. A total of 84.8 percent of patients had their follow-up visit within 72 hours of discharge. Of patients who passed the 30-day measure (Depression-T15b), 96.9 percent had their first follow-up within 14 days of discharge and 98.8 percent within 21 days. There is some controversy about including in the numerator a follow-up visit that occurred on the same day as hospital discharge. Computing the scores for this measure while requiring a follow-up on post-discharge Day 1 or later resulted in only slightly lower seven-day and 30-day rates: 78.9 percent and 93.9 percent, respectively.

Comparative Results from Other Sources

Follow-up after Hospitalization for Mental Illness (Depression-T15a, Depression-T15b). The percentage with follow-up after hospitalization for mental health conditions is well documented among multiple insurance plans, patient populations, and health systems. For patients in commercial, Medicaid, and Medicare HMO plans in 2014,

Table 5.17
Depression Measure Scores Related to Follow-up After Hospitalization for Mental Illness, 2013–2014

Measure	Numerator[a]	Denominator[a]	Measure Score (%)
Percentage of psychiatric hospital discharges among patients with depression with follow-up within			
• seven days [Depression-T15a]	3,231	3,709	87.1
• 30 days [Depression-T15b]	3,532	3,709	95.2

[a] Based on administrative data; direct and purchased care.

the follow-up visit scores are 53.0, 43.9, and 35.3 percent, respectively, within seven days of MH-related discharge, and 71.0, 63.0, and 54.3 percent, respectively, within 30 days (National Committee for Quality Assurance, 2015b). For those in commercial or Medicare PPO plans in 2014, follow-up visit scores are 49.6 and 34.7, respectively, within seven days of MH-related discharge, and 69.2 and 56.7 percent, respectively, within 30 days (National Committee for Quality Assurance, 2015b). An evaluation of VHA mental health services found 45.8 and 78.1 percent of patients with depression in FY 2007 received a follow-up visit within seven and 30 days of MH-related hospital discharge, respectively (Sorbero et al., 2010). Among a sample of veterans discharged from a psychiatric inpatient stay with an MDD diagnosis between 2004 and 2008 (n = 45,587), 39.4 percent had a follow-up visit within seven days of discharge, and 75.8 percent received follow-up within 30 days (Pfeiffer et al., 2011). In a review of MHS care delivered in 2013, percentages with follow-up care after discharge from MH-related hospitalizations were 58.5 percent within seven days and 74.8 percent within 30 days for direct care, and 34.4 percent within seven days and 57.4 percent within 30 days for those with purchased care (DoD, 2014c). The MHS measure scores from Phase I of this study were 86.2 percent and 95.1 percent (Depression-T15a, Depression-T15b, respectively) (Hepner et al., 2016). Based on 2013–2014 data in the current report, we found measure scores (87.1 and 95.2 percent, respectively) that were slightly higher than those for 2012–2013. The MHS scores on these measures continue to be substantially higher than those from other health systems. This suggests that MHS has developed a good system for follow-up care for patients with depression after MH-related hospitalization.

Quality of Care for Depression over Time and by Service Branch, TRICARE Region, and Service Member Characteristics, Based on Administrative Data

Six of seven depression measure scores increased between 2012–2013 and 2013–2014, but these increases were small (i.e., increases ranged from less than 1 to 4 percentage points). However, a small decrease was observed in the percentage with a follow-up visit within 30 days of a new antidepressant prescription for depression (Depression-T6). These results suggest a general trend of improved quality of care provided to active-component service members for depression over time.

In our previous report, we examined quality measure scores for the 2012–2013 depression cohort by service branch, TRICARE region, and service member characteristics, including age, gender, race/ethnicity, pay grade, and deployment history for the administrative data–based quality measures (Hepner et al., 2016). Several large and statistically significant differences in quality of care were observed for the depression quality measures across branches of service and TRICARE region in the 2012–2013 analyses. As with the PTSD measures, the variations in care were not consistent across measures; however, the results still raise concerns about whether care is consistent and equitable in the MHS.

We updated results for the administrative data–based quality measures using 2013–2014 data to examine whether these variations in care remained. The quality of depression care varied widely by service branch and TRICARE region. Percentages with follow-up visits within seven days of MH discharge (Depression-T15a) differed across service branches by as much as 15 percent for the depression cohort. For the depression cohort, differences in measure scores by TRICARE region were largest for receipt of a minimum of six months of antidepressant prescriptions (Depression-T5b; 9 percent) and follow-up visits within seven days of an MH-related discharge (Depression-T15a; 9 percent). We also observed significant variations in quality of depression care by service member characteristics. In the depression cohort, percentages with adequate filled prescriptions for antidepressants (Depression-T5a and Depression-T5b) varied across pay grades by up to 24 and 30 percent, respectively. The depression measure scores also exhibited wide variation by race/ethnicity and age. Percentages with adequate filled antidepressants (Depression-T5a and Depression-T5b) differed across age groups by up to 18 and 24 percent, respectively. The large observed disparities in depression measure scores by service branch, TRICARE region, and service member characteristics suggest the need for more consistency in care provided to these subgroups. A larger number of significant results were observed for differences in the measure scores for depression than PTSD (Table 4.18), although reasons for these differences are unclear.

In Table 5.18, we highlight the characteristics for which measure scores showed statistically significant variation for the depression measures. For the subgroups that exhibit statistically significant differences, additional information on the direction of the differences for each measure is detailed in Table 5.19. A set of charts showing the variation in depression measure scores by these characteristics is presented in Appendix D.

Summary

In the list below, we highlight key findings from this chapter assessing care for depression.

Depression Measures: Key Findings

- **Assessment for suicidal risk and recent substance use** occurred frequently (88–90 percent) for service members beginning an NTE for depression. This was similar to or better than other published military results.

Table 5.18
Summary of Service and Member Characteristics with Statistically Significant Differences in 2013–2014 Quality Measure Scores for Depression

Depression Measure	Service Branch	Region	Age	Race/ Ethnicity	Gender*	Pay Grade	Deployment History
New antidepressant for ≥ 12 weeks (T5a)	X	X	X	X		X	X
New antidepressant for ≥ 6 months (T5b)	X	X	X	X		X	X
Visit in 30 days after new antidepressant (T6)	X	X		X			
Psychotherapy within 4 months of NTE (T8)	X						X
Care within 8 weeks of NTE (T9)							
Visit in 7 days after MH discharge (T15a)	X	X					X
Visit in 30 days after MH discharge (T15b)	X	X					X

NOTE: X = One or more statistically significant differences (*P* < 0.05) among subgroups defined by this characteristic.

* The measure scores for T5b (new antidepressant for ≥6 months) differed significantly between males and females before the *P*-values were adjusted for multiple comparisons, but differences were not significant after the adjustment.

- **Assessment of baseline symptom severity** of depression with the PHQ-9 occurred only slightly more than a third of the time (37 percent, as represented in the medical record), although current efforts are under way within the MHS to increase the regular use of the PHQ-9 to monitor depression symptoms.
- **Assessment for behaviors of mania or hypomania** was conducted in just one-quarter (26 percent) of patients beginning a new treatment episode for depression.
- **Standardized tools** were used in less than half of the assessments for suicide risk and recent substance use, almost never used in assessment of function, and never used in assessment for behaviors of mania or hypomania.

Table 5.19
Summary of Statistically Significant Differences in 2013–2014 Quality Measure Scores, by Service and Member Characteristics for Depression

Depression Measure	Significant Results
New antidepressant for ≥ 12 weeks (T5a)	Branch: Air Force > Marine Corps/Navy > Army Region: West/Overseas/North > South Age: 45–64/35–44 > 25–34 > 18–24 Race/Ethnicity: White, non-Hispanic > Hispanic > Black, non-Hispanic; Other-Unknown > Black, non-Hispanic Pay Grade: O4–O6/O1–O3> E5–E9 > E1–E4 Deployment: Deployed > Not deployed
New antidepressant for ≥ 6 months (T5b)	Branch: Air Force > Army/Marine Corps; Navy >Army Region: West > North > South; Overseas > South Age: 45–64/35–44 > 25–34 > 18–24 Race/Ethnicity: White, non-Hispanic/Other-Unknown > Hispanic > Black, non-Hispanic Pay Grade: O4–O6/O1–O3 > E5–E9 > E1–E4 Deployment History: Deployed > Not deployed
Visit in 30 days after new antidepressant (T6)	Branch: Marine Corps/Navy > Air Force/Army Race: Other-Unknown > Black Region: Overseas > West/South; North > South
Psychotherapy within 4 months of NTE (T8)	Branch: Army > Air Force Deployment: Deployed > Not deployed
Care within 8 weeks of NTE (T9)	Scores for this quality measure showed no variation by the characteristics examined.
Visit in 7 days after MH discharge (T15a)	Branch: Air Force/Army > Marine Corps/ Navy Region: South/West/Overseas > North Deployment: Deployed > Not deployed
Visit in 30 days after MH discharge (T15b)	Branch: Army/Air Force > Marine Corps/Navy Region: South/West > North Deployment History: Deployed > Not deployed

NOTE: Comparisons between subgroups listed in this table showed a statistically significant difference at $P < 0.05$.

- Appropriate **minimal care for patients with positive suicidal ideation** was less than optimal (30 percent), primarily due to a lack of documentation regarding addressing access to lethal means. A Safety Plan Worksheet has recently been added to the clinical guideline for assessment and management of suicide risk which may improve this performance in the future.
- Adequate **duration of new antidepressant treatment** was 65 percent for the acute phase (i.e., 12 weeks) and 46 percent for the continuation phase (i.e., six months), similar to or better than other comparative scores. Fewer (41 percent) had an **evaluation and management visit** within 30 days of a newly prescribed antidepressant.
- Most depression patients with an NTE (56 percent) had at least one **psychotherapy** session in the first four months of care. Among all who received psycho-

therapy, 30 percent received any therapy that included at least two components of CBT.

- A low proportion (25 percent) of depression patients beginning an NTE received an adequate amount of **care (either psychotherapy or evaluation and management visits) in the eight weeks following the start of an NTE**.
- Rates of minimal **utilization of the PHQ-9** showed continuous increase over the three four-month intervals (34, 40, and 51 percent), though the rate of re-measurement at five to seven months for those with a PHQ-9 score greater than 9 was 38 percent. Rates of **response and remission** based on PHQ-9 scores were low (7 percent and 4 percent, respectively).
- **Follow-up after hospitalization for a mental health diagnosis** continued to be very high among patients with depression compared with other health care settings, with 87 percent seen within seven days and 95 percent within 30 days.
- Comparing **results over time**, six of seven depression measure scores increased between 2012–2013 and 2013–2014, but these increases were small (i.e., less than 1 to 4 percentage points). However, a small decrease was observed in the percentage of having a follow-up visit within 30 days of a new antidepressant prescription.
- Comparing **measure scores by service characteristics**, scores by service branch differed up to 15 percent for follow-up after mental health discharge. Scores by TRICARE region differed up to 9 percent for two measures: a minimum of six months of antidepressant prescriptions and follow-up after mental health discharge.
- Comparing **measure scores by member characteristics**, scores by pay grade differed up to 30 percent for adequate filled prescriptions for antidepressants. Scores by age groups differed up to 24 percent also for adequate filled prescriptions for antidepressants.

At the time of the publication of this report, the updated CPG for MDD was released (U.S. Veterans Administration and DoD, 2016). The updated CPG supports the content of the quality measures reported here for depression, specifically, careful initial assessment, assessment and follow-up for suicide risk, monthly monitoring after the initiation of care (pharmacotherapy and/or evidence-based therapy), and regular use of the PHQ-9 to assess progress.

CHAPTER SIX

Use of Symptom Questionnaires and Relationship Between Evidence-Based Care and Symptom Scores

In this chapter, we present preliminary analyses of clinical outcomes for service members who receive treatment for PTSD or depression in the MHS and explore the link between guideline-concordant care and outcomes. The analyses presented in this chapter focus on symptom questionnaire data collected through the BHDP. The BHDP is a secure web-based system for collecting behavioral health symptom data directly from MHS patients, which has been in operation since September 2013 in all of Army's behavioral health clinics. Implementation of the BHDP is still in the early stages in Navy and Air Force BH clinics. More detail about this unique data source is provided in Chapter Two. We restricted all analyses of symptom questionnaire data in this chapter to Army personnel in the PTSD and depression cohorts defined in Chapter Two (Methods) of this report. Personnel in the Navy, Air Force, and Marines were not included in any of these analyses due to the limited use of the BHDP system by other service branches in 2013–2014. Analyses in Chapters Four and Five were restricted to those who received only direct care, whereas in this chapter we examine symptom scores for those who received any direct mental health specialty care during the 12-month observation period. Mental health specialty visits are defined to include outpatient visits with specific codes based on the MEPRS code–3rd level variable in the CAPER outpatient file.[1] In addition, it is important to point out that the analyses in Chapter Six are unrelated to measures PTSD-T1 (Table 4.18) and Depression-T1 (Table 5.18), which are a measurement of minimal utilization (at least one symptom score during a four-month interval if any condition-related encounter occurred).

We focused the analyses in this chapter on two symptom scores. The PCL scores were analyzed for soldiers in the PTSD cohort. MEDCOM Policy 14-094 (Department of the Army Headquarters, 2014b) requires the frequency of administration of the PCL to be every 30 days for soldiers. Of the 10,045 Army personnel in the PTSD cohort, 28 and 18 percent have a follow-up PCL score 60 to 120 days and five to

---

[1] The following codes for outpatient care are included in the definition of mental health specialty care: BFA (psychiatry clinic), BFB (psychology clinic), BFD (mental health clinic), BFE (social work clinic), BFF (outpatient social work clinic), BFZ (psychiatric care, not elsewhere classified).

seven months from the first PCL score in their observation window, respectively.[2] The PHQ-9 scores were analyzed for soldiers in the depression cohort. The recommended frequency of the PHQ-9 is as follows: "at every clinical encounter where a depressive disorder is the focus of treatment. At a minimum, the PHQ-9 should be administered upon treatment initiation and at least once between 60–120 days after intake" (DoD, 2014e). Of the 16,980 Army personnel in the depression cohort, 18 and 12 percent have a follow-up PHQ-9 score 60 to 120 days and five to seven months from the first PHQ-9 score in their observation window, respectively.[3] It is important to point out that these analyses are unrelated to measures PTSD-T10 and -T12 (Table 4.18) and Depression-T10 and -T12 (Table 5.18), which are a measurement of follow-up of elevated scores (remeasurement five to seven months after a score at or above a triggering threshold with a condition-related encounter).

While the primary purpose of analyzing these symptom scores was to explore whether increased receipt of guideline-concordant care predicted improved treatment outcomes, we also conducted descriptive analyses in order to understand how these two symptom questionnaires in BHDP are used by Army behavioral health providers. In this chapter, we present analyses that describe Army's implementation of outcome monitoring using BHDP. We describe the number of completed symptom questionnaires for patients relative to how many mental health specialty visits they have had during the 12-month observation period. To assess whether those who complete symptom questionnaires differ from those who do not, we compare the characteristics of Army personnel with those who completed one symptom questionnaire or none, among the subgroup of soldiers with at least two mental health specialty visits.

Following the descriptive analyses, we present analyses of the symptom scores using multivariable regression models to address specific questions. To measure change in the symptom scores over time after controlling for the potential effects of other variables, we fit repeated measures multivariable linear regression models to initial and six-month symptom scores for each service member. To evaluate whether receiving guideline-concordant care, as assessed by administrative data-based quality measures, was associated with improvement in symptom scores from the initial score to six months, we conducted a set of analyses of the symptom scores, controlling for other variables using multivariable regression models. We analyzed the follow-up symptom scores completed five to seven months after the initial score to be consistent with the six-month time period used in the quality measures for response and remission based

---

[2]   These scores are not related to those reported in Table 4.18 (Chapter Four) for measure PTSD-T1, a measurement of minimal utilization (at least one PCL score during a four-month interval if any PTSD-related encounter occurred) and not a measurement of follow-up.

[3]   These scores are not related to those reported in Table 5.18 (Chapter Five) for measure Depression-T1, which is a measurement of minimal utilization (at least one PHQ-9 score during a four-month interval if any depression-related encounter occurred) and not a measurement of follow-up.

on symptom questionnaire data. For a detailed description of these analyses, see Chapter Two.

At the end of the chapter, we examine whether the overall monthly completion of symptom questionnaires (for PCLs in the PTSD cohort, and for PHQ-9s in the depression cohort) increased over time within the Army in 2013–2014, relative to the overall monthly number of behavioral health specialty visits completed by those in the PTSD and depression cohorts, respectively.

Completion of Symptom Questionnaires by Army Personnel

Implementation of the BHDP system within the Army has been targeted toward behavioral health clinics. Therefore, it would be expected that only patients with at least one mental health specialty visit would complete these questionnaires. This is the pattern we observed in an analysis that included all Army personnel in the PTSD cohort (n = 10,045).[4] As expected, among Army soldiers in the PTSD cohort without any mental health specialty care visits at an MTF in 2013–2014, very few completed a PCL during their 12-month observation period (Figure 6.1). Of the Army person-

Figure 6.1
Percentages of Army Personnel in PTSD Cohort with No, One, or Two or More PCL Scores, by Number of Mental Health Specialty Visits in Direct Care, 2013–2014

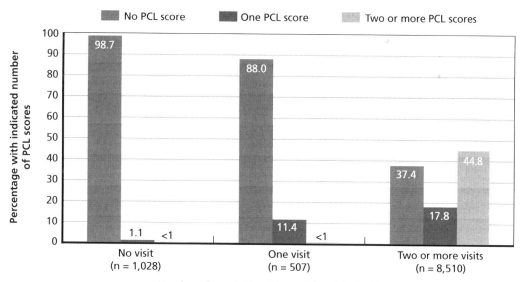

RAND RR1542-6.1

---

[4] A detailed description of the eligibility criteria for the PTSD cohort is provided in Chapter Two (Methods) in this report. Briefly, the cohort includes active-component service members who received care for PTSD and are engaged with and eligible for MHS care.

nel in the PTSD cohort who had only one mental health specialty care visit, most did not complete any PCLs; about one in ten completed one PCL, and only a few completed two PCLs. Few patients may complete a PCL at the first specialty care visit for two reasons. First, patients complete an intake questionnaire at the first specialty care visit. Second, the provider must update the symptom questionnaire frequency in BHDP for ongoing outcome monitoring, a task typically completed after the patient has received a psychiatric diagnosis. In contrast, among Army personnel who had two or more mental health specialty care visits, close to half completed two or more PCLs during the 12-month observation period. Yet, even among this group with two or more mental health specialty visits, over a third did not complete any PCLs.

A similar pattern of PHQ-9 completion was observed in an analysis of all Army personnel in the depression cohort (N = 16,980; see Figure 6.2).[5] As expected, of Army personnel in the depression cohort with no mental health specialty care visits in 2013–2014, almost none completed a PHQ-9 during the 12-month observation period. Of Army personnel in the depression cohort who had only one mental health specialty care visit, fewer than one in ten completed a PHQ-9. In contrast, among Army personnel who had two or more mental health specialty care visits, one-third completed

Figure 6.2
Percentages of Army Personnel in Depression Cohort with No, One, or Two or More PHQ-9 Scores, by Number of Mental Health Specialty Visits in Direct Care, 2013–2014

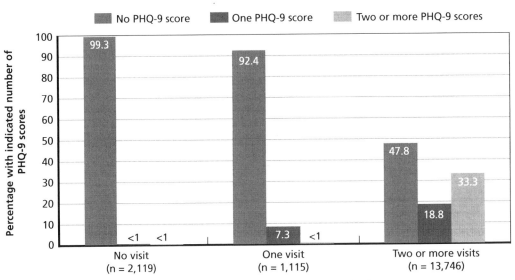

RAND RR1542-6.2

[5]   A detailed description of the eligibility criteria for the depression cohort is provided in Chapter Two (Methods) in this report. Briefly, the cohort includes active-component service members who received care for depression and are engaged with and eligible for MHS care.

two or more PHQ-9s during their 12-month observation period, but almost half did not complete any PHQ-9s. Notably, fewer soldiers in the depression cohort completed two or more PHQ-9s than what was observed for completion of PCLs by soldiers in the PTSD cohort.

Comparing Army Personnel Who Completed Two or More Symptom Questionnaires with Those Who Completed One or None

In this section, we compare the service member and treatment characteristics of Army personnel in the PTSD (or depression) cohort who completed two or more symptom questionnaires during the 12-month observation period with a combined group of those who completed one questionnaire and those who did not complete any questionnaires. These analyses are limited to Army personnel who have two or more mental health specialty visits, to increase the likelihood that we focus on soldiers whose behavioral health outcomes are most likely to be monitored with symptom questionnaires. These analyses provide a preliminary assessment of whether any variations existed in the implementation of BHDP, and whether those who completed at least two symptom questionnaires differ from those who completed one symptom questionnaire or none. It should be noted that any variation related to service member characteristics or their treatment could be related to variation in local Army BHDP implementation or in service members' willingness to complete the symptom questionnaires. When the BHDP is used consistently by all providers in all mental health specialty clinics, the pattern of these results may change.

The first set of comparisons focused on the completion of the PCL by the PTSD cohort. This analysis included the 8,510 Army personnel in the PTSD cohort with two or more mental health visits at MTFs in 2013–2014, representing 84.7 percent of the 10,045 Army personnel in the PTSD cohort. Of the 8,510 Army personnel, 3,815 (44.8 percent) completed two or more PCLs during the 12-month observation period (Figure 6.1); this group was compared with those who filled out one PCL or none (n = 4,695). There were significantly different distributions by pay grade and region of those in the PTSD cohort who completed two or more PCLs than of those completing one PCL or none (Table 6.1). The differences are likely due to different rollout schedules and levels of implementation across regions throughout 2013–2014. In addition, significantly more of those completing two or more PCLs used inpatient care (28.5 versus 19.2 percent) and also had more outpatient visits for any reason (median number 58 versus 37) and for mental health specialty visits (median number 24 versus 11 among those with at least two) (Table 6.2).

The second set of comparisons focused on the completion of the PHQ-9 by the depression cohort. This analysis included the 13,746 Army personnel in the PTSD cohort with two or more mental health visits in MTFs in 2013–2014, representing

Table 6.1
Member and Service Characteristics, by Number of Completed PCLs, Among Army Personnel in PTSD Cohort with Two or More Mental Health Specialty Visits in MTFs in 12-month Observation Period, 2013–2014

Characteristic	Percentage with Zero or One PCL Score (n = 4,695)	Percentage with Two or More PCL Scores (n = 3,815)	P-value
Gender			
Female	15.8	14.3	NS
Male	84.2	85.7	
Race/ethnicity			
White, non-Hispanic	57.4	56.1	NS
Black, non-Hispanic	21.9	23.2	
Hispanic	13.8	13.2	
Other/unknown	6.9	7.6	
Age			
18–24	12.6	12.3	NS
25–34	45.0	47.1	
35–44	35.4	34.7	
45 and over	6.9	6.0	
Pay grade			
E1–E4	25.3	26.7	0.0072
E5–E9	63.8	64.5	
O1–O3	3.8	3.3	
O4–O8	4.6	3.2	
Warrant	2.6	2.3	
Years of service			
0–3	9.5	9.4	NS
4–6	17.1	17.9	
7–10	23.7	25.7	
11–15	21.5	21.1	
16–20	20.0	17.8	
More than 20	8.2	8.1	

Table 6.1—Continued

Characteristic	Percentage with Zero or One PCL Score (n = 4,695)	Percentage with Two or More PCL Scores (n = 3,815)	P-value
Never deployed[a]	6.6	5.9	NS
Region			
North	13.6	20.3	< 0.0001
Overseas	9.6	15.1	
South	37.5	38.2	
West	35.9	25.0	
Unknown	3.4	1.4	

NOTE: NS = not significant.

[a] Based on data from September 2001 through March 2015.

Table 6.2
Health Care Utilization, by Number of Completed PCLs, Among Army Personnel in PTSD Cohort with Two or More Mental Health Specialty Visits in MTFs in 12-month Observation Period, 2013–2014

Characteristic	Zero or One PCL Score (n = 4,695)	Two or More PCL Scores (n = 3,815)	P-value
Percentage of patients with any acute inpatient care	19.2	28.5	< 0.0001
Median number of outpatient visits, any diagnosis (among those with at least one outpatient visit, any diagnosis)	37	58	< 0.0001
Median number of outpatient MH specialty visits (among those with at least two outpatient MH specialty visits)	11	24	< 0.0001

81.0 percent of the 16,980 Army personnel in the depression cohort. Of the 13,746 Army personnel in the depression cohort with two or more mental health visits in 2013–2014, 33.3 percent (n = 4,588) completed two or more PHQ-9s during the time period (Figure 6.2); this group was compared to those who filled out one PHQ-9 or none (n = 9,158). In the depression cohort, the distributions of those completing two or more PHQ-9s differed significantly from those completing one PHQ-9 or none for gender, race/ethnicity, pay grade, deployment, and region (Table 6.3). Similar to PCL completion, the differences in PHQ-9 completion are likely due to different rollout schedules and levels of implementation across regions throughout 2013–2014. In addition, significantly more of those completing two or more PHQ-9s used inpatient care (30.0 versus 22.2 percent), and they also received more outpatient visits for any reason

Table 6.3
Member and Service Characteristics, by Number of Completed PHQ-9s, Among Army Personnel in Depression Cohort with Two or More Mental Health Specialty Visits in MTFs in 12-month Observation Period, 2013–2014

Characteristic	Percentage with Zero or One PHQ-9 Score (n = 9,158)	Percentage with Two or More PHQ-9 Scores (n = 4,588)	P-value
Gender			
Female	29.6	26.5	0.0002
Male	70.4	73.5	
Race/ethnicity			
White, non-Hispanic	58.0	55.1	0.0124
Black, non-Hispanic	23.4	25.4	
Hispanic	12.2	12.9	
Other/unknown	6.4	6.6	
Age			
18–24	21.8	20.6	NS
25–34	44.2	44.8	
35–44	28.1	29.5	
45–64	5.9	5.1	
Pay grade			
E1–E4	39.1	39.8	< 0.0001
E5–E9	48.4	51.7	
O1–O3	5.2	3.9	
O4–O8	5.2	3.1	
Warrant	2.1	1.6	
Years of service			
0–3	21.9	20.8	NS
4–6	20.8	20.4	
7–10	20.4	21.8	
11–15	16.2	16.8	
16–20	14.8	14.2	
More than 20	5.9	5.9	

Table 6.3—Continued

Characteristic	Percentage with Zero or One PHQ-9 Score (n = 9,158)	Percentage with Two or More PHQ-9 Scores (n = 4,588)	P-value
Never deployed[a]	23.6	20.7	0.0001
Region			
North	19.3	21.2	< 0.0001
Overseas	11.2	14.5	
South	32.3	38.0	
West	34.4	25.2	
Unknown	2.8	1.2	

[a] Based on data from September 2001 through March 2015.

Table 6.4
Health Care Utilization, by Number of Completed PHQ-9s, Among Army Personnel in Depression Cohort with Two or More Mental Health Specialty Visits in MTFs in 12-month Observation Period, 2013–2014

Characteristic	Zero or One PHQ-9 Score (n = 9,158)	Two or More PHQ-9 Scores (n = 4,588)	P-value
Percentage of patients with any acute inpatient care	22.2	30.0	< 0.0001
Median number of outpatient visits, any diagnosis (among those with at least one outpatient visit, any diagnosis)	33	52	< 0.0001
Median number of outpatient MH specialty visits (among those with at least two outpatient MH specialty visits)	9	22	< 0.0001

(median number 52 versus 33) and for mental health specialty visits (median number 22 versus 9 among those with at least two) (Table 6.4).

Examining Change in Symptom Scores Between Initial Score and Six Months Later

We examined whether PCL and PHQ-9 scores significantly changed over the six months following the initial score for the PTSD and depression cohorts, respectively. According to the Working Group's recommendations, PTSD (or depression) patients seen in the behavioral health clinics should have been reminded to complete a PCL (or PHQ-9) "at the initiation of treatment and as clinically indicated during treatment (preferably at each treatment session), but at least once between 60–120 days after intake" (DoD, 2014e). As described in Chapter Two, we analyzed data on the sample of service members having initial and six-month symptom scores. The initial score in our analyses was defined as the first symptom score after the individual enters the PTSD (or depression) cohort.[6] We did not require a "clean period," that is, a period of time before the initial score, to verify that it was associated with the first treatment of PTSD (or depression) ever or for a specified minimum period of time. For the follow-up score, if there were multiple scores in the five-to-seven-month period, the last one in the window was selected.

Since follow-up scores were not available for every soldier in the PTSD cohort who received at least one mental health specialty care visit, we weighted the data for those having follow-up scores to obtain results representative of the PTSD (or depression) cohort obtaining direct mental health specialty care having at least one visit. In other words, with respect to observed characteristics, soldiers with initial and six-month symptom scores who are more similar to those without both scores were weighted more heavily in the analysis than those who were less similar. As described in Chapter Two, the weights adjusted for differences between those with versus without follow-up scores with respect to age (18–24, 25–34, 35–44, 45 and older), male (0,1), race/ethnicity (white, non-Hispanic; black, non-Hispanic; Hispanic; other), pay grade (E1–E4, E5–E9, O1–O3, O4–O8), region (north south, west, overseas), Charlson comorbidity index, and number of years of service. Those with an initial score and follow-up score in the five-to-seven-month window represented 19.5 percent (1,762/9,017) of Army personnel in the PTSD cohort with one or more mental health specialty visits in MTFs and 13.5 percent (2,009/14,861) of Army personnel in the depression cohort with one or more mental health specialty visits in MTFs. Furthermore, those with a follow-up score in the five-to-seven-month window represented 46.2 percent (1,762/3,815) of Army personnel in the PTSD cohort with two or more PCL scores, and 43.8 percent (2,009/4,588) of Army personnel in the depression cohort with two or more PHQ-9 scores. The logistic regression output for the models predicting the probabilities of having a six-month score after the initial score, which are inverse weights for the analyses for each cohort, are provided in Appendix E (Tables E.1 and E.3 for the PTSD and depression cohorts, respectively).[7] Table E.1 shows that, for the PTSD cohort, having higher Charlson comorbidity index scores[8] and being male were significantly associated

---

[6]   A detailed description of the eligibility criteria for the PTSD (or depression) cohort is provided in Chapter Two (Methods) in this report. Briefly, the cohort includes active-component service members who received care for PTSD (or depression) and are engaged with and eligible for MHS care.

[7]   Appendixes for this report are available online: http://www.rand.org/pubs/research_reports/RR1542.html.

[8]   Indicators were created for 17 medical conditions, using diagnosis codes and procedure codes from inpatient and outpatient claims data. The Charlson comorbidity index score is a weighted sum of those indicators.

with having a follow-up PCL score, and there was significant variation across regions with respect to having follow-up PCL scores. Table E.3 shows that, for the depression cohort, there were significant associations between pay grade and region with the probability of having a follow-up score. The weighting adjusts the analysis results for these differences so that results represent the population of those receiving at least one direct mental health specialty care visit.

Table 6.5 shows the average initial and six-month symptom scores for each cohort, along with symptom change scores, adjusted for service member characteristics. For each cohort, the results are presented for four subsets: All service members; those with high initial symptom scores (50 or higher); those in an NTE; those with high initial symptom scores (50 or higher) and in an NTE.

In the PTSD cohort, the average initial PCL score was 55 for all service members, indicating the initial scores were above the PTSD score associated with a diagnosis (i.e.,

Table 6.5
Six-month Change in Symptom Scores Among Army Personnel in the PTSD and Depression Cohorts Receiving Mental Health Specialty Care in MTFs, Adjusted for Service Member Characteristics, 2013–2014

	N[a]	Initial Score (standard error)	Six-month Score (standard error)	Adjusted Change Score (standard error)[b]	t-statistic	P-value
PCL Score in PTSD Cohort						
All	1,762	54.91 (0.35)	53.36 (0.37)	−1.55 (0.32)	−4.81	< 0.0001
Those with initial PCL ≥ 50	1,127	63.44 (0.28)	58.75 (0.41)	−4.69 (0.38)	−12.49	< 0.0001
Those with an NTE	289	54.02 (0.84)	51.06 (0.95)	−2.96 (0.74)	−3.98	< 0.0001
Those with initial PCL ≥ 50 and an NTE	186	62.13 (0.66)	56.58 (1.10)	−5.55 (0.89)	−6.21	< 0.0001
PHQ-9 Score in Depression Cohort						
All	2,009	15.57 (0.13)	13.82 (0.14)	−1.75 (0.14)	−12.69	< 0.0001
Those with initial PHQ-9 ≥ 10	1,731	17.10 (0.10)	14.75 (0.15)	−2.35 (0.15)	−16.08	< 0.0001
Those with an NTE	455	15.41 (0.27)	13.19 (0.30)	−2.22 (0.29)	−7.60	< 0.0001
Those with initial PHQ-9 ≥ 10 and an NTE	389	16.98 (0.22)	14.14 (0.31)	−2.84 (0.31)	−9.19	< 0.0001

NOTE: PTSD and depression cohorts are not mutually exclusive.

[a] The analysis sample consists of service members having both initial and 6-month symptom scores. The sample is weighted to reflect the population of service members receiving any direct mental health specialty care.

[b] The change score estimate is adjusted for the following service member characteristics: Charlson comorbidity index, number of years in service, age, sex, race/ethnicity, pay grade, and region.

50). The average decrease in PCL scores over six months was 1.55 points. However, the average decreases were greater for the subsets of service members with high initial PCL score (i.e., 50 or higher) and/or- in an NTE (Table 6.5). The greatest point decrease (-5.55 points) was for those with both an NTE and an initial score of 50 or above. The average decrease for those in the PTSD cohort with an initial PCL score of 50 or above was 4.69 points. All of these decreases are far below the reductions in scale scores of 10 to 20 points that are considered clinically meaningful change (Monson et al., 2008). Of those with initial PCL scores of at least 50, at six months 2 percent had remission (PCL < 28), 46 percent had at least a 5-point reduction, and 39 percent had higher symptom scores.

In the depression cohort, the average initial PHQ-9 score was 16 for the analysis of all eligible service members, indicating moderately severe depression. The average decrease in PHQ-9 scores over six months was 1.75 points. As with the PTSD cohort, the average reductions in PHQ-9 scores were greater for those with relatively high initial PHQ-9 scores and/or NTEs. For example, those with an initial PHQ-9 score of 10 or greater and in an NTE had an average decrease of 2.84 points. A five-point (or greater) change in PHQ-9 scores reflects clinically significant change (Löwe et al., 2004). However, the reductions in PHQ-9 scores reported in Table 6.5 for the various subgroups of the depression cohort did not achieve this magnitude of change. Among those with initial PHQ-9 scores of at least 10 points, 5 percent achieved remission (PHQ-9 < 5), 14 percent had a 50-percent reduction in PHQ-9 scores from their initial score, and 40 percent had higher symptom scores. Full regression model output for the analyses estimating the change scores is provided in Appendix E (Tables E.2, E.4, and E.18–E.23).

Examining the Relationship Between Guideline-Concordant Care and Improved Outcomes

Next, we examined whether receipt of care specified by each quality measure was associated with a change in six-month symptom scores. We also examined whether a composite measure summarizing receipt of some portion of the care specified by the four (for PTSD) or five (for depression) administrative data–based quality measures was associated with a change in six-month symptom scores. We focused on the administrative data–based measures in these models because they allowed us to maximize the sample sizes included in the multivariate analyses, compared with the much smaller samples included in the medical record measures. The symptom questionnaire measures could not be used because they are measuring change in the same symptom scores (i.e., PCL and PHQ-9) as the models. These analyses focused on those service members with initial and six-month symptom scores. Average initial PCL scores significantly differed (mean = 53.5 points) for those whose last observed symptom scores were either in the zero-to-four-month window (mean = 54.9 points) or in the eight-to-12-month window (mean = 53.5 points) (P = 0.0092). Average initial PHQ-9 scores (mean = 15.6 points) statistically significantly differed from those whose last observed symptom scores were either in the zero-to-four-month window (mean = 15.2 points) or eight-to-12-month window (mean = 15.7 points) (P = 0.0216).

Analyses were weighted to represent the population of service members eligible to receive at least one of the quality measures. Weighting was specific to each cohort (i.e., PTSD or depression). The logistic regression output for the models predicting the probabilities of having an initial and six-month score, inverse weights for the analyses for each cohort, are provided in Appendix E (Tables E.5 and E.6) for the PTSD and depression cohorts, respectively. The results show that most member and service characteristics examined were not significantly associated with having initial and six-month scores. However, region and Charlson comorbidity index scores were significantly associated with having initial and six-month scores in both the PTSD and depression cohorts. Regional differences could arise from implementation progressing at different rates at different MTFs, and a higher comorbidity index indicates sicker people receive more care. In the PTSD cohort, more years of service and pay grade were associated with having initial and six-month scores. More time in the service could lead to more deployments and more exposure to trauma. The weighting adjusted the analysis results for these differences.

The tests of association of the quality measures and change in symptom scores are presented in Table 6.6 for the PTSD cohort and Table 6.7 for the depression cohort. Full regression model output for the analyses is provided in Appendix E (Tables E.7–E.11 and E.12–E.17) for PTSD and depression cohorts, respectively. As Tables 6.6 and 6.7 show, receipt of guideline-concordant care, as assessed by the quality measures, was not significantly associated with changes in symptom scores.

Change Over Time in Completion of PCL and PHQ-9

To characterize how the use of the BHDP changed over time for Army soldiers within our cohorts, we estimated symptom questionnaire completion rates for PCLs in the PTSD cohort and PHQ-9s in the depression cohort on a monthly basis in 2013–2014. It is worth noting that the period covered by our analysis (January 2013 through June 2014) started only four months after the use of BHDP was mandated for all routine individual behavioral health care in Army behavioral health clinics by the U.S. Army Medical Command (MEDCOM) Operations Order (OPORD) 12-47 (dated August 30, 2012) (U.S. Army Task Force on Behavioral Health, 2013). MEDCOM Policy 14-094 (Department of the Army Headquarters, 2014b) requires the frequency of administration of the PCL to be every 30 days for soldiers. For each month in Figure 6.3, we limited the analysis to Army personnel in the PTSD cohort who had two or

Table 6.6
Six-month Adjusted Change in PCL Scores Associated with Receipt of Care Indicated by the PTSD Quality Measures Among Army Personnel Receiving Mental Health Specialty Care, PTSD Cohort, 2013–2014

PTSD Quality Measure[a]	n[b]	PCL Mean Initial Score (standard error)	PCL Adjusted Change (standard error)[c]	t-statistic	P-value
New SSRI/SNRI for ≥ 60 days (T5)	378	55.8 (0.75)	−0.95 (1.39)	−0.68	0.4943
Visit in 30 days after new SSRI/ SNRI (T6)	374	55.93 (0.75)	1.86 (1.35)	1.38	0.1692
Psychotherapy within 4 months of NTE (T8)	285	53.83 (0.50)	0.68 (2.02)	0.34	0.7362
Care within 8 weeks of NTE (T9)	273	53.95 (0.88)	−0.72 (1.64)	−0.44	0.6627
Composite measure[d]	572	55.01 (0.62)	0.37 (0.73)	0.51	0.6077

[a] See Appendix A for detailed technical specifications for the PTSD quality measures.

[b] The analysis sample consists of service members having both initial and 6-month symptom scores. The sample is weighted to reflect the population of service members receiving any direct mental health specialty care.

[c] The change score estimate is adjusted for the following service member characteristics: initial symptom score, Charlson comorbidity index, number of years in the service, age, sex, race/ethnicity, pay grade, and region.

[d] The PCL Adjusted Change estimate for the composite measure is scaled to reflect the expected change in PCL scores for Army personnel who receive all recommended care in the set of the other four measures shown in the table.

more direct care mental health specialty visits from January 2013 through the month before the "index month." For example, for the completion rate in May 2014, we limited the analysis to the 12,356 Army personnel in the PTSD cohort who had two or more direct care mental health specialty visits in the period from January 2013 through April 2014. For those 12,356 personnel, we counted the number of PCLs they completed during May 2014 (n = 1,867), and their number of mental health specialty visits during May 2014 (n = 9,216). We calculated the "PCL completion rate" for May 2014 as the number of completed PCLs per 100 mental health specialty visits (1,867/9,216, or 20.3 PCLs per 100 mental health specialty visits). The number of mental health specialty visits on which these rates are based increased from 8,727 in February 2013 to a high of 15,684 in July 2013 and gradually decreased to 8,487 in June 2014.[9] Over the same period, the number of completed PCLs on which the rates are based increased

---

[9]   The large decrease in the number of mental health specialty visits from July 2013 (15,684/24,709 for PTSD/ depression cohorts) to June 2014 (8,487/13,650) is due to the method we used to estimate the rates of completion. We limited the analysis to service members in the PTSD and depression cohorts identified between January and June 2013, resulting in an initial increase in the number of MH specialty visits from February 2013 to July 2013 as the number of service members in the cohorts increased, and then a decrease in the number of mental health

Table 6.7
Six-month Adjusted Change in PHQ-9 Scores Associated with Receipt of Care Indicated by the Depression Quality Measures Among Army Personnel Receiving Mental Health Specialty Care, Depression Cohort, 2013–2014

Depression Quality Measure[a]	n[b]	PHQ-9 Initial Score (standard error)	PHQ-9 Adjusted Change (standard error)[c]	t-statistic	P-value
New antidepressant for ≥ 12 weeks (T5a)	594	15.81 (0.23)	−0.80 (0.56)	−1.43	0.1539
New antidepressant for ≥ 6 months (T5b)	588	15.81 (0.23)	−0.78 (0.49)	−1.58	0.1140
Visit in 30 days after new antidepressant (T6)	582	15.79 (0.24)	−0.11 (0.47)	−0.24	0.8111
Psychotherapy within 4 months of NTE (T8)	444	15.41 (0.27)	−0.84 (0.64)	−1.31	0.1894
Care within 8 weeks of NTE (T9)	420	15.35 (0.28)	−0.15 (0.56)	−0.27	0.7881
Composite measure[d]	823	15.68 (0.22)	−0.48 (0.27)	−1.78	0.0751

[a] See Appendix B for detailed technical specifications for the depression quality measures.

[b] The analysis sample consists of service members having both initial and 6-month symptom scores. The sample is weighted to reflect the population of service members receiving any direct mental health specialty care.

[c] The change score estimate is adjusted for the following service member characteristics: initial symptom score, Charlson comorbidity index, number of years in the service, age, sex, race/ethnicity, pay grade, and region.

[d] The PHQ-9 Adjusted Change estimate for the composite measure is scaled to reflect the expected change in PHQ-9 scores for Army personnel who receive all recommended care in the set of the other four measures shown in the table.

from 424 in February 2013 to 1,825 in June 2014. The PCL completion rate increased from 4.9 per 100 visits in February 2013 to 21.5 per 100 visits in June 2014. This suggests that the completion of PCLs by Army personnel in the PTSD cohort increased about fourfold from January 2013 to June 2014.

We repeated the same steps for Army personnel in the depression cohort by counting the number of mental health specialty visits and PHQ-9s in each month from February 2013 through June 2014. We found the PHQ-9 completion rate for the depression cohort increased over time (Figure 6.3) at a rate similar to PCL completion in the PTSD cohort. The symptom questionnaire completion rate for PHQ-9s in the depression cohort increased from 3.1 per 100 visits in February 2013 to 17.2 per 100 visits in June 2014. The number of mental health specialty visits on which these PHQ-9 rates are based increased from 12,481 in February 2013 to a high of 24,709

specialty visits beginning in July 2013 and continuing through June 2014 as the use of care by the cohort members decreased over time.

Figure 6.3
Symptom Questionnaire Completion Rate, by Cohort and Month, Army Personnel, February 2013–June 2014

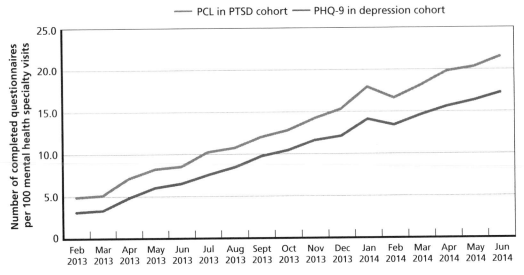

NOTE: PTSD and depression cohorts are not mutually exclusive.
RAND RR1542-6.3

in July 2013, and gradually decreased to 13,650 in June 2014. Over the same period, the number of completed PHQ-9s increased from 392 in February 2013 to 2,343 in June 2014. Figure 6.3 also shows that the completion rate is consistently higher for the PTSD cohort than for the depression cohort.

These completion rate analyses were limited to soldiers who have had at least two direct mental health specialty care visits and excluded those with only one mental health specialty visit. The analyses also included only patients who received a PTSD (or depression) diagnosis in January to June 2013 and therefore were eligible for the PTSD (or depression) cohort. These restrictions may mean these completion rates are not representative of all soldiers receiving care in BH clinics.

Limitations of the Symptom Questionnaire Data and Analyses

As described in Chapter Two, these data and analyses have limitations. Because the BHDP data represent only a subset of the service members with PTSD or depression, conclusions based on symptom questionnaire data collected through the BHDP should be interpreted cautiously and may not apply to the group as a whole. Several characteristics may differ between those with symptom scores and those without. Importantly, the data in our analyses are limited to Army personnel. In addition, at the time of this study, scores from symptom questionnaires completed by patients seen for psychological health conditions in primary care within the MTFs or by patients with visits for psychological health conditions with primary care or mental health specialty providers outside of MTFs (i.e., purchased care) were not typically included in the BHDP data. Scores from symptom questionnaires completed in primary care within the MTFs could be entered into data-mineable fields in AHLTA, but these would not be captured in BHDP and were not included in these analyses. In addition, examining whether there are associations between quality measures and symptom scores requires risk adjustment in order to account for the possibility that receiving the indicated care is associated with preexisting condition severity. Failure to risk adjust could lead to biased tests of association. The regression and weighting adjustments we used for the multivariate analyses adjust for known patient characteristics, such as demographics and initial symptom scores. However, our analyses do not account for unobserved or unrecorded differences, so our results would be biased if such factors exist and are important. Another limitation, as discussed above, is that the initial score in our analyses may not be a "true baseline," in that we do not require a "clean period," that is, a period of time before the initial score to verify that it was associated with the first treatment of PTSD (or depression) ever or for a specified minimum period of time. When restricting the analyses of change in symptom scores to those with a new treatment episode and/or clinically meaningfully high symptom scores, we estimated larger reductions in symptoms. However, these analyses are prone to the possibility of regression-to-the-mean bias, in which measurements that are extreme on their first measurement will tend to be closer to average on subsequent measurement (Bland and Altman, 1994). Also, we assessed the association between individual process measures and one composite of the process measures in the regression analyses. Alternative approaches to developing and scoring composites could be evaluated in future analyses. Finally, some MTF providers and clinics do not yet use BHDP consistently.

Summary

Since 2012, Army behavioral health clinics have collected standardized symptom questionnaires using the BHDP. Army intends to use these symptom score data to inform both clinical care and assessment of patient outcomes. Of the 8,510 Army personnel in our PTSD cohort who had two or more mental health specialty care visits, 45 percent completed two or more PCLs over their 12-month observation period in 2013–2014, but only 1,762 had an initial score and a score five to seven months later. Of the 13,746 Army personnel in the depression cohort who had two or more mental health specialty care visits, one-third completed two or more PHQ-9s in their 12-month observation period, but only 2,009 had an initial score and a score five to seven months later. A few differences in service member and treatment characteristics between those completing two or more questionnaires and those who completed one questionnaire or none were statistically significant in both the PTSD and depression cohorts. Although these differences were small with regard to most characteristics examined, those with two or more questionnaires were much higher users of inpatient and outpatient care than those who completed one questionnaire or none.

We also conducted preliminary analyses to examine whether treatment outcomes, as measured by symptom questionnaires from BHDP, improved from the initial score (i.e., the first score observed) to six months later among Army soldiers with two or more mental health specialty visits. These multivariate analyses adjusted for service member characteristics. In the PTSD cohort, the average decrease in PCL scores from the initial score to six months was 1.55 points, while in the depression cohort, the average decrease in PHQ-9 scores over six months was 1.75 points. Both changes were statistically significant, although changes of this magnitude would not be considered clinically meaningful. While these preliminary analyses may accurately reflect that soldiers who receive at least two visits of mental health specialty treatment do not achieve clinically meaningful improvement six months later, it is important to use caution in interpreting these results. However, the average decreases were greater for the subsets of service members with initial symptom scores that were relatively high and/ or in an NTE. The data reflect a subset with continued engagement and reassessment in behavioral health specialty care. Those having multiple behavioral health specialty care visits may respond or remit in less than five months and would not be reflected in these results. To explore this, we conducted sensitivity analyses (not shown) examining outcomes at two to four months. Average reductions in symptom scores were less than or similar to those reported here for the five-to-seven-month analyses. We weight our analysis results to account for our reliance on an opportunistic assessment of those remaining in care. However, the weights adjust only for observed initial characteristics, so it is possible that our findings could be biased by adverse selection of a sample having the most severe/chronic conditions, if such selection is not accounted for by the characteristics used to weight the data. However, the mean initial symptom scores by time of last recorded symptom score were statistically significantly different, though they differed by 1.5 points at most. Specifically, mean initial PCL scores for those with their last PCL observed at zero to four months was 53.5 points; for those with a follow-up score in the five-to-seven-month window it was 54.9 points; and those without a PCL in the five-to-seven-month window but with their last PCL in eight to 12 months was 53.5 points ($P = 0.0216$). For PHQ-9, these estimates were 15.2, 15.6, and 15.7, respectively ($P = 0.0092$). For both cohorts, results were significantly lower for those with the last observation in the zero-to-four-month window versus in the five-to-seven-month window ($P < 0.05$ in both cohorts). More work is needed to understand whether particular subgroups demonstrate clinically meaningful improvement within six months (e.g., service members with more severe symptoms at the time of the initial score). Similarly, significant predictors of improvement could be identified that could guide approaches to improving treatment outcomes (e.g., number of visits, type of treatment). At a minimum, these results suggest that more analyses of service member outcomes are needed to assess the effectiveness of treatment delivered by the MHS.

In another set of multivariate models, we found no significant associations between receiving the guideline-concordant care, as specified in the PTSD and depression quality measures, and improvements in patient symptom scores at six months after the initial score. There are two possible limitations to the generalizability of these findings. First, the sample is small and is based on those with new episodes of care or beginning medication treatment. Second, our analyses could be subject to bias from unobservable factors, and our weights account only for observed baseline characteristics. Although each of these quality measures has face validity because they measure key aspects of clinical practice guidelines, demonstrating predictive validity can be useful in identifying the most important process of care measures (McGlynn and Adams, 2014). Despite many efforts to demonstrate predictive validity for individual quality measures, this has proven difficult, and there remain few empirical studies that demonstrate a significant association between process of care measures and improvements in clinical outcomes for mental health conditions (Hepner et al., 2007; Parast et al., 2015). The administrative data quality measures examined in this chapter, along with the measures described in Chapters Four and Five that did not have a sufficient number of service members to include in multivariate analyses, still provide useful information about the quality of care delivered to service members with PTSD or depression.

We assessed the use of the BHDP for completing the PCL and PHQ-9 on a monthly basis from February 2013 through June 2014. We found the overall PCL completion rate in the PTSD cohort and overall PHQ-9 completion rate in the depression cohort increased steadily in 2013–2014 to 21.5 and 17.2 per 100 MH specialty visits, respectively, in June 2014. Although these rates are relatively low, they represent a time period early in the use of the BHDP system when providers and patients were new to the system, and completion rates would be expected to continue to increase over time. Notably, the completion rate was consistently higher for the PCL by the PTSD cohort than for the PHQ-9 for the depression cohort throughout the entire period.

Finally, while the analyses presented in this chapter are preliminary, they demonstrate the potential value of routinely collected data on patient outcomes. The Army's use of BHDP as a measurement-based care tool for clinicians also provides valuable data to track patient outcomes across the Army and at local MTFs. These data can provide ongoing feedback on whether patients receiving care in the MHS are improving, and more detailed analyses can target treatment approaches to improve outcomes. As the implementation of BHDP continues enterprise-wide, these data will provide similarly useful information for other service branches.

CHAPTER SEVEN

Summary and Recommendations

In this chapter, we highlight the strengths and limitations of the analyses in this report, summarize areas in which the MHS performs well and areas which represent a priority for improvement efforts, and present policy recommendations and directions for future research. We identified cohorts of active-component service members who received care for PTSD and depression from the MHS (direct or purchased care) in 2013–2014. Allowing a six-month time frame in 2013 for cohort entry, we identified almost 15,000 and over 30,000 active-component service members who received treatment for PTSD and depression, respectively, from the MHS. We described the characteristics of these service members and the types of services received, the providers seen, and the treatment settings where care was delivered. Further, we characterized the quality of care these patients received for these two conditions using a set of quality measures based on administrative data, medical record data, and symptom questionnaire data. Finally, we explored the symptom questionnaire data available from the BHDP for Army personnel to document patterns of completion of the PCL and PHQ-9 and examined the change in symptom scores over time and the relationship between the symptom scores and guideline-concordant care.

Strengths of the Analyses

The analyses presented in this report have several strengths.

- We present an enterprise view of the care provided to the PTSD and depression cohorts, including all direct care and purchased care during 2013–2014.
- We also present measure scores for a set of quality measures during that same period.
- We use data from three different sources with unique strengths:
  - Administrative data: These data are readily available and comprehensive in that they include all TRICARE encounters, both direct and purchased care.
  - Medical record data: These data provide a level of clinical detail not available from other data sources. Because the MHS uses a common electronic health

record, all outpatient direct care regardless of specialty is documented in a
single medical record.

- Symptom questionnaire data: These data are relatively easy to access and provide a source of patient self-reported symptoms over time.
- The results in this report provide a set of administrative data measures from 2013–
2014 that can be compared to the results from 2012–2013 in our previous report.
- We also present analyses utilizing medical record data and symptom questionnaire data that the MHS can use to monitor changes over time in the quality of
care provided.

Limitations of the Analyses

The work presented in this report also has several limitations. These limitations are
related to the potential for inherent error in the data and the variable coverage of the
different sources in terms of which service members were included.

- Administrative data: These data were used to assign patients to the PTSD and
depression cohorts and summarize aspects of care received. We may have inappropriately included or missed patients based on provider use of diagnosis codes.
We also required just one visit or inpatient stay with a PTSD or depression diagnosis for cohort entry (if other cohort requirements were met). We chose to require
one encounter to be more inclusive but acknowledge that we may have included
patients whose diagnosis was not confirmed. On the other hand, requiring only
one encounter meant that we were also not excluding those patients with a valid
diagnosis who may not have received indicated follow-up care. When we computed scores for selected measures, both with denominators that required just one
study condition diagnosis and more than one diagnosis, the computed results
revealed little difference between the two measure scores. Another limitation is
that multiple records in the administrative data may be associated with a single
health care encounter. Translation of these data into discrete inpatient stays and
outpatient encounters is challenging. Based on a detailed review of the data available to us, we created rules to increase the likelihood that inpatient and outpatient
encounters were counted appropriately and quality measures applied in a manner
that adhered to detailed specifications. Despite these efforts, there may be unin-
tended variation in the classification of the administrative data. Also, we cannot
account for visits that may have been inappropriately coded with regard to the
care received. Evaluation of other important aspects of care delivery, such as the
impact of an integrative or collaborative care models, are beyond the scope of this
project, as they are difficult to accurately characterize using administrative data.

- Medical record data: The only source of outpatient medical record data available to this study was AHLTA. This meant that our MRR sample was limited to those active-component service members who received direct care only during the 12-month observation period. As a data source, MRR data are also time and budget intensive to access, which resulted in our needing to reduce the amount of MRR data we could collect for this study. Also, any care received that was not documented in the record would not have been included in our analyses. In addition, even when a central electronic health record is utilized, in some cases a "shadow record" (separate paper document) may exist that would not be accessible to the medical record abstractor.

- Symptom questionnaire data: We restricted all analyses of symptom questionnaire data to Army personnel in the PTSD and depression cohorts. In addition, the samples for the symptom questionnaire quality measures in Chapters Four and Five are further restricted to Army personnel with one or more symptom questionnaires who used *direct care only* during the 12-month observation period. Personnel in Navy, Air Force, and Marines were not included in any of these analyses due to the limited use of the BHDP system by other service branches in 2013–2014. In addition, symptom questionnaires are typically not completed within BHDP by patients seen in primary care for psychological health conditions within the MTFs or by patients with visits for psychological health conditions with primary care or mental health specialty providers outside of MTFs (i.e., purchased care). Therefore, these data are not representative of all service members in the PTSD and depression cohorts.

- We were unable to compare direct care and purchased care due to the small percentage of service members who obtained purchased care exclusively.

- We excluded service members who failed to meet eligibility requirements from our cohorts (41 percent of those potentially eligible for the PTSD cohort and 35 percent of those potentially eligible for the depression cohort).[1] That failure suggests that they separated from the military during their observation year. Those who were excluded had higher average initial PCL and PHQ-9 scores (for PCL, 56.2 versus 53.3 points, $p < 0.0001$; for PHQ-9, 16.3 versus 15.3 points, $p < 0.0001$). Further work is needed to understand the characteristics and care received for service members who separate within a year following a diagnosis of PTSD or depression.

- The depression quality measures presented here were applied to patients with a diagnosis of depression (MDD or other depression diagnosis). This definition of depression was used to accommodate the variable ICD-9 code definitions of MDD and depression as used in some NQF-endorsed quality measures. However, the CPG VA and DoD, 2009) specifically targets patients with a diagnosis of

---

1   Only 3 to 5 percent of those potentially eligible (PTSD and depression, respectively) were excluded by reason of deployment.

MDD rather than just any depression. Therefore, there is a need to validate some of the measures applied here. However, the just-published update of the MDD CPG recommends considering its principles when treating other depressive disorders, in particular, unspecified depressive disorders (VA and DoD, 2016).

- A final limitation is related to the set of quality measures we present. The focus of these measures is outpatient care. Therefore, important aspects of care that occurred in the inpatient setting are not included in this evaluation. In addition, most of the depression measures are more established than the PTSD measures, with published results from other health care systems. Six of the depression measures (addressing suicide screening, antidepressant treatment, use of the PHQ-9, response to treatment, remission of symptoms, and follow-up of psychiatric hospitalization) are NQF-endorsed, but only one of the PTSD measures (follow-up of psychiatric hospitalization) is. Thus, the PTSD measures will require additional testing and validation, and comparison to other populations as data become available.

Despite these limitations, this report provides a comprehensive, enterprise view of service members who receive care for PTSD or depression and an assessment of the care they receive across several quality measures. The remainder of this chapter highlights the main findings from the report, followed by the policy implications of the findings.

Main Findings

Service Members with PTSD or Depression Have a High Level of Health Care Services Utilization with Multiple Providers, Suggesting the Need to Ensure Effective Coordination of Care

Service members in the PTSD and depression cohorts were frequent users of inpatient and outpatient care, when considering care for both medical and psychiatric conditions. For example, one in five patients in both cohorts had an inpatient hospitalization. Service members in the PTSD and depression cohorts had a median of 40 and 31 outpatient visits for any reason during the 12-month observation period, respectively. The median number of visits with PTSD or depression as the primary diagnosis was ten visits and four visits, respectively. Furthermore, they saw many different providers for their outpatient care (i.e., a median of 14 and 12 unique providers during the 12-month observation period for service members in the PTSD and depression cohort, respectively). We found high percentages of comorbid PH conditions in both cohorts. While our analyses of visits and providers included both medical and psychiatric care, we did not examine medical comorbidities. Although some patients are receiving a large volume of medical care, the care provided is not always what is recommended by clinical practice guidelines, as evidenced by their low percentages of receiving adequate initial treatment for PTSD and depression—36 percent and 25 percent, respectively, of patients in a new treatment episode had four psychotherapy visits or two evaluation and management visits within eight weeks. These findings suggest there is much to be learned about patterns of care provided to service members with PTSD and depression, and how that care is coordinated.

Many Service Members with PTSD or Depression Receive Multiple Psychotropic Medications Including Some High-Risk Medications, Suggesting the Need for Quality Monitoring

Many service members with PTSD or depression received four or more psychotropic medications (45 percent of the PTSD cohort and 32 percent of the depression cohort). A third of PTSD patients and a quarter of depression patients filled at least one prescription for a benzodiazepine. About 57 percent of PTSD patients and 50 percent of depression patients filled at least one prescription for an opioid. These findings suggest the need for more extensive analyses of these prescribing patterns to understand their rationale and to develop and apply strategies for quality monitoring.

Quality Measures for PTSD and Depression Identified Both Strengths and Areas for Improvement

We examined the quality of care for PTSD and depression over 12 months using several quality measures. Measure scores above 75 percent were considered to be high and those below 50 percent were considered to be low, although published scores for the same or similar measures in comparable populations also informed our assessment. While it is often difficult, or not appropriate, to directly compare results from other health care systems or studies or related measures, prior results were presented to provide context to guide interpretation of the results. In Table 7.1, we provide an overview of measure scores, similar to the dashboard we provided in our Phase I report (Hepner et al., 2016). In general, there is a trend of better performance on PTSD measures than on the depression measures. Based on our consideration of available contextual data from other sources, the clinical importance of the process (e.g., related to suicide risk), and significant variation across service branch or TRICARE region, we highlight areas of strength for the MHS in green and areas that may be high priorities for improvement in yellow. For measures not highlighted, we were not able to make this assessment, typically due to lack of contextual data. Readers are encouraged to review the detailed results for each measure presented in Chapters Four and Five. It should be noted that the MHS should work toward maintaining high performance or improving on all of these measures. Nonetheless, this summary provides a preliminary dashboard to guide further quality improvement efforts for PH conditions. We provide further discussion of these results in the next sections.

Table 7.1
Overview of Quality Measure Results for PTSD and Depression

PTSD		Depression	
	PTSD		**Depression**
Measure	**Score (%) (denominator)**	**Measure**	**Score (%) (denominator)**
Assessment: Symptom Severity and Comorbidity			
Percentage of PTSD patients with a new treatment episode with assessment of symptoms with PCL [PTSD-A1]	46.7 (229)	Percentage of depression patients with a new treatment episode with assessment of symptoms with PHQ-9 [Depression-A1]	37.2 (234)
Percentage of PTSD patients with a new treatment episode assessed for depression [PTSD-A2]	93.9 (229)	Percentage of depression patients with a new treatment episode assessed for manic/ hypomanic behaviors [Depression-A2]	25.6 (234)
Percentage of PTSD patients with a new treatment episode assessed for suicide risk [PTSD-A3]	96.1 (229)	Percentage of depression patients with a new treatment episode assessed for suicide risk[a] [Depression-A3]	87.6 (234)[b]
Percentage of PTSD patients with a new treatment episode assessed for recent substance use [PTSD-A4]	93.0 (229)	Percentage of depression patients with a new treatment episode assessed for recent substance use [Depression-A4]	90.2 (234)
Treatment: Follow-up for Suicidal Ideation			
Percentage of patient contacts of PTSD patients with SI with appropriate follow-up (PTSD-T3)	54.2 (24)	Percentage of patient contacts of depression patients with SI with appropriate follow-up (Depression-T3)	30.2 (53)
Treatment: Medication Management			
Percentage of PTSD patients with a newly prescribed SSRI/SNRI with an adequate trial (≥60 days) [PTSD-T5]	72.7 (2,547)	Percentage of depression patients with a newly prescribed antidepressant with a trial of:	
		• 12 weeks[a] [Depression-T5a]	65.3 (8,314)
		• Six months[a] [Depression-T5b]	46.0 (8,222)
Percentage of PTSD patients newly prescribed an SSRI/SNRI with follow-up visit within 30 days [PTSD-T6]	44.6% (2,539)	Percentage of depression patients newly prescribed an antidepressant with follow-up visit within 30 days [Depression-T6]	41.3% (8,216)
Treatment: Psychotherapy			
Percentage of PTSD patients who receive evidence-based psychotherapy for PTSD [PTSD-T7]	45.3 (351)	Percentage of depression patients who receive evidence-based psychotherapy for depression [Depression-T7]	29.9 (345)
Percentage of PTSD patients with a new treatment episode who received any psychotherapy within four months [PTSD-T8]	74.1 (2,600)	Percentage of depression patients with a new treatment episode who received any psychotherapy within four months [Depression-T8]	56.2 (7,225)

Table 7.1—Continued

PTSD		Depression	
Measure	Score (%) (denominator)	Measure	Score (%) (denominator)
Treatment: Receipt of Care in First Eight Weeks			
Percentage of PTSD patients with a new treatment episode with 4 psychotherapy visits or 2 E&M visits within the first 8 weeks [PTSD-T9]	35.5 (2,608)	Percentage of depression patients with a new treatment episode with 4 psychotherapy visits or 2 E&M within the first 8 weeks [Depression-T9]	25.1 (7,009)
Treatment: Symptom Assessment and Response to Treatment			
Percentage of PTSD patients with symptom assessment with PCL during 4-month measurement period [PTSD-T1]		Percentage of depression patients with symptom assessment with PHQ-9 during 4-month measurement period[a] [Depression-T1]	
• Months 1–4	44.0 (2,697)	• Months 1–4	33.5 (2,329)
• Months 5–8	51.3 (1,578)	• Months 5–8	40.4 (1,298)
• Months 9–12	62.0 (1,343)	• Months 9–12	51.3 (1,157)
• Overall	50.4 (5,618)	• Overall	39.7 (4,784)
Percentage of PTSD patients (PCL score > 43) with response to treatment (5-point reduction in PCL score) at 6 months [PTSD-T10]	18.7 (916)	Percentage of depression patients (PHQ-9 score > 9) with response to treatment (50% reduction in PHQ-9 score) at 6 months[a] [Depression-T10]	7.1 (770)
Percentage of PTSD patients (PCL score > 43) in PTSD-symptom remission (PCL score <28) at six months [PTSD-T12]	1.2 (916)	Percentage of depression patients (PHQ-9 score > 9) in depression-symptom remission (PHQ-9 score < 5) at six months[a] [Depression-T12]	3.5 (770)
Percentage of PTSD patients with a new treatment episode with improvement in functional status at six months [PTSD-T14]	NR (229)	Percentage of depression patients with a new treatment episode with improvement in functional status at six months [Depression-T14]	NR (234)
Treatment: Psychiatric Discharge Follow-up			
Percentage of psychiatric inpatient hospital discharges of patients with PTSD with follow-up in		Percentage of psychiatric inpatient hospital discharges of patients with depression with follow-up in:	
• Seven days[a] [PTSD-T15a]	87.6 (1,859)	• Seven days[a] [Depression-T15a]	87.1 (3,709)
• 30 days[a] [PTSD-T15b]	96.1 (1,859)	• 30 days[a] [Depression-T15b]	95.2 (3,709)

NOTES: Green indicates areas of strength for the MHS, while yellow indicates areas that may be high priorities for improvement. PTSD and depression cohorts are not mutually exclusive.

[a] NQF-endorsed measure.

[b] Denominator includes additional depression codes besides MDD. Score for NQF-endorsed version is similar but applies to fewer patients.

The MHS Continues to be a Leader in Achieving High Scores for Follow-up After Psychiatric Hospitalization

Our results replicate our prior findings and provide additional support that the MHS has achieved high percentages with follow-up of active-component service members in the PTSD and depression cohorts after a hospitalization with a mental health diagnosis. The percentages with follow-up after psychiatric hospitalization were markedly higher relative to other health care systems (within seven days: 88 percent for PTSD; 87 percent for depression; within 30 days: 96 percent for PTSD; 95 for depression). Earlier in this report, we highlighted policy memos that may have played a key role in achieving this performance. For example, one memo described follow-up procedures for missed behavioral health appointments, including those after mental health hospital discharges (Department of the Army Headquarters, 2011). Another emphasized the need for follow-up within the first 72 hours after discharge, including avoidance of weekend and federal holiday discharges to support this effort (Department of the Army Headquarters, 2014a). Further investigation to better understand how these high percentages of follow-up were achieved would be useful in developing quality improvement efforts for enhancing follow-up and care coordination in other contexts. We note that there is still variation in these measure scores across service branch (up to 14 percentage points in variation), highlighting the need to ensure consistent performance.

The MHS Performed Well in Providing Initial Screening for Suicide and Substance Abuse But Needs to Improve at Providing Adequate Follow-up to Service Members with Suicide Risk

Our results suggest that the MHS demonstrates relatively high performance in providing screening for suicide risk for service members beginning a new treatment episode for PTSD or depression (96 percent for PTSD; 88 percent for depression). Similarly, the MHS appears to perform well in conducting screening for some comorbid disorders in these patients. Measure scores for comorbid substance use screening were 93 percent for PTSD and 90 percent for depression, while screening for comorbid depression in patients with PTSD was 94 percent. Screening for manic or hypomanic behaviors in patients with a new episode of depression, however, was just 26 percent, suggesting this may be an area for improvement. Note that we did not assess whether there was appropriate follow-up to address the comorbid condition if identified (e.g., substance use disorder [SUD]).

Providing adequate follow-up for service members who screen positive for suicide risk is a high priority area for improvement for the MHS. Because DoD/VA CPG on suicide risk (VA and DoD, 2013) may not have been fully implemented in clinical practice at the time of our medical record review, we chose to apply a minimal level of follow-up to those patients with SI not hospitalized in response to the SI. Minimal follow-up required an assessment for plan and means, a referral or follow-up appointment, and a discussion of limiting access to lethal means or documentation of no access to lethal means. Almost all nonhospitalized patients with SI were seen by behavioral health providers, were assessed for presence or absence of a suicide plan, and were given referrals or follow-up appointments that were usually complied with in the one to two weeks after the visit. However, the score for the suicide follow-up measure was 54 percent for PTSD and 30 percent for depression. These scores were primarily the result of a lack of documentation in the medical record addressing lethal means. Since this study was initiated, a Safety Plan Worksheet (VA, 2014), which incorporates limitation of access to lethal means, was added to the 2013 CPG for suicide risk management. Generalized use of this tool could facilitate improved performance of this measure in the future.

Given these results and the published CPG, the MHS has an opportunity to strengthen its approach to the delivery of care for those presenting with positive SI.

The MHS Continues to Have Moderately Low Scores for Providing Adequate Initial Care and Follow-up for Service Members Beginning Treatment for PTSD or Depression

The MHS continued to demonstrate relatively low scores of providing adequate initial treatment for PTSD and depression—36 percent and 25 percent, respectively, had four psychotherapy visits or two E&M visits within eight weeks of a new treatment episode. These scores suggest the MHS could improve on providing treatment to service members when they are starting treatment, as indicated by at least six months without any treatment for the condition. Similarly, we found that the MHS could improve at providing timely follow-up when service members are beginning a new prescription treatment for PTSD or depression. Less than half (45 percent) of those in the PTSD cohort and 41 percent in the depression cohort had a medication management visit in the 30 days after newly prescribed medication treatment.

Most Service Members with PTSD or Depression Received at Least Some Psychotherapy, But the MHS Could Increase Delivery of Evidence-Based Psychotherapy

Our descriptive analyses once again demonstrated that a very high proportion of patients in both cohorts received at least one psychotherapy visit (i.e., individual, group, or family therapy) during their observation period—over 90 percent of the PTSD cohort and nearly 85 percent of the depression cohort. This represents a slight increase from the prior year (2012–2013 scores were 90 percent and 81 percent). Furthermore, service members in the PTSD and depression cohorts with any psychotherapy received a notably high average number of therapy visits at 18.6 and 14.3, respectively, of which 14.6 and 8.6 visits on average were associated with the primary cohort diagnosis. These levels of psychotherapy utilization are higher than those reported in the civilian sector. A study of psychotherapy utilization among a sample of privately insured patients found 74.6 percent and 62.4 percent of PTSD and MDD patients, respectively, received any psychotherapy visits during calendar year 2005 (Harpaz-Rotem, Libby, and Rosen-heck, 2012). Harpaz-Rotem and colleagues found that PTSD patients received 12.6 therapy visits, and MDD patients completed 9.9 visits, on average. This suggests there is notably higher therapy initiation and engagement among PTSD and depression patients within the MHS than among those in the civilian health care sector.

In our assessment of the quality of psychotherapy delivered, results suggest that the MHS could increase delivery of guideline-concordant psychotherapy. Among service members who received psychotherapy, 45 percent and 30 percent received any therapy that appeared consistent with evidence-based therapy (at least two components documented in the medical record, in at least one session) within the PTSD and depression cohorts, respectively.

Army Increased Outcome Monitoring, But Improvements Are Still Needed in Rates of Outcome Monitoring and Performance on Outcome Measures

The Army has shown leadership in advancing the effort to monitor outcomes among patients seen in behavioral health specialty care using symptom questionnaire data collected through the BHDP. The BHDP has provided a source of accessible data based on symptom questionnaires completed by patients, including (but not limited to) the PCL and PHQ-9. At the time of this data collection, the BHDP had not yet extended beyond Army behavioral health care. However, the BHDP provided us with an opportunity to use this source of data to compute scores for measures related to monitoring symptoms and response to treatment within six months. Although the data were limited to Army direct behavioral health care, they provide some insight about symptom monitoring and response to care for service members seen in these treatment settings. Assessment of symptoms with the PCL for PTSD and PHQ-9 for depression showed increasing performance over the 12-month observation period (44 to 62 percent for PTSD and 34 to 51 percent for depression). Response to treatment and remission were evaluated among those patients with a score of a particular threshold (i.e., greater than 43 for the PCL and greater than 9 for the PHQ-9) within six months. Response (i.e., five-point PCL score reduction or 50 percent PHQ-9 reduction) was 19 percent for PTSD and 7 percent for depression. Remission (PCL score less than 28 or PHQ-9 score less than 5) was very low, at 1 percent for PTSD and 4 percent for depression. Improvement in function within six months of a new PTSD or depression diagnosis could not be assessed due to the lack of use in the studied population of standardized tools to evaluate this outcome. These results represent an initial assessment of patient outcomes and highlight the importance of ongoing monitoring of outcome measures. The current expansion in the MHS of the use of the BHDP across the service branches will provide an opportunity to monitor these measures enterprise-wide.

In examining changes in symptom scores over time, we found that symptom scores improved from the initial score to six months later among Army soldiers with two or more mental health specialty visits by a statistically significant, but not a clinically meaningful, amount for the group as a whole. However, the average reductions were greater for the subsets of service members with initial relatively high symptom scores and/or in a new treatment episode. We did not detect significant associations between receiving recommended care, as specified in the PTSD and depression quality measures, and improvements in patient symptoms at six months after the initial score. Finally, while these analyses are preliminary, they demonstrate the potential value of routinely collected data on patient outcomes. More research on particular subgroups may demonstrate clinically meaningful improvement within six months (e.g., service members with more severe symptoms at the time of the initial score).

Administrative Data–Based Quality Measures Suggest Care for PTSD and Depression Improved Slightly Between 2012–2013 and 2013–2014

Examining performance for the same quality measures in 2012–2013 and 2013–2014, we found five of the six PTSD scores for measures based on administrative data increased less than 1 to 3 percentage points between the two time periods. The largest of these increases related to having at least 60 days of an SSRI/SNRI filled prescription. However, one measure score decreased less than 1 percentage point over this time period: the percentage with a follow-up visit within 30 days of a new SSRI/SNRI prescription for PTSD. Six of seven depression measure scores also increased between 2012–2013 and 2013–2014, but the sizes of these increases were less than 1 to 4 percentage points. A decrease of less than 1 percentage point was observed in the percentage with a follow-up visit within 30 days of a new antidepressant prescription for depression. These results suggest a general trend of improved quality of care provided to active-component service members for PTSD and depression over time. Over such a short time frame and without any targeted efforts for improvement in these measures, large changes in measure scores would not be expected. It was outside the scope of this project to identify and describe quality improvement efforts over this same period.

Quality of Care for PTSD and Depression Varied by Service Branch, TRICARE Region, and Service Member Characteristics, Suggesting an Opportunity for Further Learning About Underlying Reasons for These Variations

Using 2013–2014 administrative data, we conducted an assessment of the variation in measure scores by service branch, TRICARE region, and service member characteristics, including age, gender, race/ethnicity, pay grade, and deployment history, as we had conducted on 2012–2013 administrative data. The largest differences occurred by branch of service, TRICARE region, pay grade, and age. For branch of service, follow-up within seven days after a mental health hospitalization (T15a) varied by up to 16 percent and 15 percent in the PTSD and depression cohorts, respectively. For TRICARE region, follow-up within 30 days after a new prescription of SSRI/SNRI (PTSD-T6) varied up to 12 percent in the PTSD cohort. For pay grade, percentages with adequate filled prescriptions for SSRI/SNRI for PTSD (PTSD-T5) and antidepressants for depression (Depression-T5a and -T5b) varied by up to 8, 24, and 30 percent, respectively. For age, percentages with adequate filled prescriptions for SSRI/ SNRI for PTSD (PTSD-T5) and antidepressants for depression (Depression-T5a and -T5b) varied by up to 10, 18, and 24 percent, respectively. The performance of the depression measures suggests even more variation across subgroups than the PTSD measures, although reasons for this are unclear. Given these extensive differences based on service branch, TRICARE region, pay grade, and age, understanding the underlying reasons for this variation is an essential first step in systematically designing quality improvement approaches.

Policy Implications

Recommendation 1. Improve the Quality of Care Delivered by the Military Health System for Psychological Health Conditions by Immediately Focusing on Specific Care Processes Identified for Improvement

The results presented in this report, combined with the results presented in the Phase I report (Hepner et al., 2016), represent perhaps the largest assessment of quality of care for PTSD and depression for service members ever conducted. We replicated results for administrative data–based quality measures shown in our prior report and expanded our analyses of quality of care to additional measures and new data sources for service members with PTSD or depression. We identified that while there are key strengths in some areas, quality of care for psychological health conditions delivered by the MHS should be improved. For example, a quarter of service members with depression and just over a third with PTSD received enough treatment when beginning a new episode of treatment (defined as four psychotherapy visits or two E&M visits within eight weeks following an initial diagnosis). Further, more patients should receive a follow-up medication management visit following the receipt of a new medication for PTSD or depression. This suggests that MHS should identify procedures that would ensure service members receive an adequate intensity of treatment and follow-up when beginning treatment. These strategies include ensuring adequate appointment availability and outreach to minimize no-shows. Implementation of collaborative care models could provide a framework to support these strategies and ongoing quality improvement. For example, recent data suggest that a stepped, centrally assisted collaborative care model for PTSD and depression (referred to as STEPS-UP) evaluated in the MHS led to increased receipt of mental health services and modest improvements in treatment outcomes (Belsher et al., 2016; Engel et al., 2016). Further, although the MHS performed well at screening for suicide risk, improvements are needed in providing adequate follow-up for those with suicide risk. For example, 30 percent of service members beginning a new treatment episode for depression who were identified as having suicide risk received adequate follow-up. Providing appropriate follow-up care for suicide risk is an essential strategy in reducing the rate of suicide among service members. Finally, given the extensive and complex patterns of psychopharmacologic prescribing, further analysis of these patterns and development and implementation of quality monitoring and improvement strategies would be valuable.

Recommendation 2. Expand Efforts to Routinely Assess Quality of Psychological Health Care

Recommendation 2a. Establish an Enterprise-Wide Performance Measurement, Monitoring, and Improvement System That Includes High-Priority Standardized Measures to Assess Care for Psychological Health Conditions

Currently, there is no coordinated enterprise-wide (direct and purchased care) system for monitoring the quality of PH care. A separate system for PH is not required; high-priority PH measures could be integrated into an enterprise-wide system that assesses care across medical and psychiatric conditions. The review of the MHS (DoD, 2014c) highlighted the need for such a system as well. Although the quality measures presented in this report highlight areas for improvement, quality measures for other PH conditions should be considered for reporting (e.g., care for alcohol use disorders). Furthermore, an infrastructure is necessary to support the implementation of quality measures for PH conditions on a local and enterprise-wide basis, and to support other activities, including monitoring performance, conducting analysis of performance patterns, validating the process-outcome link for each measure, and evaluating the effect of quality improvement strategies. This function could be executed by a DoD center focused on psychological health (e.g., DCoE) or additional psychological health quality measures could be integrated into ongoing efforts conducted by DoD Health Affairs.

Recommendation 2b. Routinely Report Quality Measure Scores for PH Conditions Internally, Enterprise-Wide, and Publicly to Support and Incentivize Ongoing Quality Improvement and Facilitate Transparency

Routine internal reporting of quality measure results (MHS-wide and at the service and MTF level) provides valuable information to identify gaps in quality, target quality improvement efforts, and evaluate the results of those efforts. The MHS is implementing quality improvement strategies using an "enterprise management approach" and "defining value from the perspective of the patient," including use of systems-approach interventions such as case managers to coordinate care (Woodson, 2016). Analyses of variations in care across service branches, TRICARE regions, or patient characteristics can also guide quality improvement efforts. While VHA and civilian health care settings have used monetary incentives for administrators and providers to improve performance, the MHS could provide special recognition in place of financial incentives or provide additional discretionary budget to MTFs for improved performance or maintaining high performance. In addition, reporting of selected quality measures for PH conditions could be required under contracts with purchased care providers (Institute of Medicine, 2010). Quality measures are an essential component of alternative payment models, such as value-based purchasing.

Reporting quality measure results externally provides transparency, which encourages accountability for high-quality care. External reporting could be focused on a more limited set of quality measures that are most tightly linked with outcomes or reported by other health care systems, while a broader set of measures that are descriptive or exploratory could be reported internally. In addition, external reporting allows comparisons with other health care systems that report publicly (though appropriate risk-adjustment is required for outcome measures). Finally, external reporting allows the MHS to demonstrate improvements in performance over time to multiple stakeholders, including service members and other MHS beneficiaries, providers, and policymakers.

In 2016, the MHS and the Defense Health Agency (DHA) launched a public, online quality reporting system (http://www.health.mil/Military-Health-Topics/Access-Cost-Quality-and-Safety) with measure scores by MTF for measures of patient safety, health care outcomes, quality of care, and patient satisfaction and access to care (Military Health System and Defense Health Agency, 2016). The set of HEDIS outpatient measures displayed on the site includes one PH measure: follow-up within seven days and 30 days after mental health discharge. The set of ORYX inpatient measures displayed on the site includes two PH measures: substance use and tobacco treatment. This system could be expanded to include other PH measures and coordinated enterprise-wide for monitoring the quality of all direct and purchased care. These are promising efforts that the MHS should continue to expand.

Recommendation 3. Expand Efforts to Monitor and Use Treatment Outcomes for Service Members with Psychological Health Conditions

Recommendation 3a. Integrate Routine Outcome Monitoring for Service Members with PH Conditions as Structured Data in the Medical Record as Part of a Measurement-Based Care Strategy

Measurement-based care has become a key strategy in the implementation of clinical programs to improve mental health outcomes (Harding et al., 2011). Evidence that feedback on patient-reported outcomes to providers actually improves patient outcomes is mixed, but suggests that feedback appears to be more effective when the data are used as part of a patient management system (Boyce and Browne, 2013). Currently, the ability to use the medical record (i.e., AHLTA) to routinely monitor clinical outcomes for patients receiving PH care in the MHS over time is limited. When clinicians assess patient symptoms or functioning using a questionnaire (e.g., PHQ-9), the resulting score may be entered as a free text note or into data-mineable fields within AHLTA. Scores entered in the text of the note (i.e., not in a structured, data-mineable field) are not easily accessible, and AHLTA does not support tracking change in symptoms over time. Routine monitoring for PTSD, depression, and anxiety disorders is now mandated by policy across the MHS (DoD, 2001) using the BHDP (DoD, 2016; DoD and VA, 2014; Department of the Army Headquarters, undated), and the service branches are working toward full implementation of this policy. While encouraging routine symptom monitoring is a positive step, the chief limitation of the BHDP is that it is not electronically linked to the medical record. As the new medical record system for the MHS is being developed, it would be advantageous to integrate outcome tracking within the medical record. Further, the MHS should explore how to obtain similar data for patients seen in purchased care.

Recommendation 3b. Monitor Implementation of BHDP Across Services and Evaluate How Providers Use Symptom Data to Inform Clinical Care

Our analyses of outcomes relied on symptom questionnaire data from the BHDP and were restricted to Army soldiers, due to Army's development and use of this tool during 2013–2014. We demonstrated the increased use of the PCL and the PHQ-9 over time among Army soldiers with PTSD or depression seen in MTF behavioral health clinics but also highlighted that data suggest that the Army can continue to increase the rates of routinely using these measures with these patients. Other service branches were using their own approaches to outcome tracking and are now migrating to BHDP. It will be essential to compute measures to document progress in the ongoing implementation of BHDP across the MHS, such as the completion rate we presented in Chapter Six. Further, it is important to understand how providers are making decisions in using the BHDP and ensure providers are able to integrate symptom questionnaire information into treatment planning and adjustment, rather than simply entering data because the MHS requires it.

Recommendation 3c. Build Strategies to Effectively Use Outcome Data and Address the Limitations of These Data

The Army's use of BHDP likely represents one of the largest efforts to capture outcomes for patients with PH conditions in the United States, and that effort should be commended. Results from the outcome quality measures provide a baseline assessment for Army MTF behavioral health clinics and suggest that efforts to monitor and improve treatment outcomes are needed. Our analyses highlighted some of the challenges of using clinic-based assessments of outcomes. A chief limitation of the BHDP is that outcome data are not collected if patients do not return to MTF specialty behavioral health care. Of those with an initial PCL score, only 32.6 percent (1,762/5,405) had a PCL score five to seven months later. Of those with an initial PHQ-9 score, only 27.6 percent (2,009/7,273) had a PHQ-9 score five to seven months later. However, mean symptom scores were only slightly lower for those with their last score recorded up to four months past their initial score. Thus, analyses of these data may be biased in the absence of these results. Our analyses did find some differences between service members who completed at least two symptom questionnaires and those who completed one symptom questionnaire or none; however, average initial symptom scores were similar. Analyses of these data should adjust for these missing data. Conducting telephone follow-up with patients who do not return to treatment would strengthen the data. Alternatively, this could be integrated into ongoing efforts to assess patient experiences in receiving care, including patient satisfaction, timeliness of care, and interpersonal quality (e.g., felt respected). Improving patient experiences in receiving care is an important outcome on its own, apart from symptom improvement. Further, the BHDP typically captures patients seen in specialty behavioral health care at an MTF and does not include patients who receive their care in primary care clinics (which frequently occurs, particularly for depression) or those who use purchased care for some or all of their care. While AHLTA includes structured, data-mineable fields to capture symptom questionnaire data, AHLTA does not easily support monitoring patient progress over time. Finding ways to collect outcome data routinely across all patients receiving care for psychological health conditions would bolster the representativeness of the data and offer a more complete picture of quality. Finally, as the MHS considers incentivizing MTFs for demonstrating improved outcomes, integrating case mix adjustment for difference in patient populations will likely be important (Kilbourne, Keyser, and Pincus, 2010; Pincus, Spaeth-Rublee, and Watkins, 2011).

Recommendation 4. Investigate the Reasons for Significant Variation in Quality of Care for PH Conditions by Service Branch, Region, and Service Member Characteristics

The variation in quality measure scores by member and service characteristics were largely unchanged from our previous 2012–2013 results (Hepner et al., 2016) to the 2013–2014 results in the current report. We found several statistically significant and clinically meaningful differences in measure scores by service branch, TRICARE region, and service member characteristics, many of which may represent clinically meaningful differences. Understanding and minimizing variations in care by personal characteristic (e.g., gender, race/ethnicity, and geographic region) is important to ensure that care is equitable, one of the six aims of quality of care improvement in the seminal report Crossing the Quality Chasm (Institute of Medicine, 2001). Exploring the structure and processes used by MTFs and staff in high- and low-performing service branches and TRICARE regions may help to identify promising improvement strategies for, and problematic barriers to, providing high-quality care (Institute of Medicine, 2001).

Directions for Future Research

The analyses presented in this report provide results that can guide the MHS in targeting efforts to improve quality of care for PTSD, depression, and other psychological health conditions. These analyses also raised several questions about the patterns of care observed and the most appropriate approaches to using the data sources included in our analyses. Here we outline several high-priority research directions, organized by data availability.

Analyses of Existing Data

Several additional analyses could be conducted using data that are readily accessible, such as administrative data and symptom questionnaire data.

- Identify predictors of high utilization, including both medical and psychiatric
- Understand prescribing patterns to identify potential problematic polypharmacy, benzodiazepine, and opioid use
- Assess longitudinal changes in quality of care in the context of MHS efforts to improve quality
- Examine variations in care to inform quality improvement and ensure care is delivered consistently to all patients
- Develop risk adjustment models (e.g., that account for differences in baseline severity and availability of follow-up questionnaire data) to support assessment of treatment outcomes using symptom questionnaire data
- Describe the care patterns for service members with PTSD or depression who eventually separated from the military or have disability claims
- Examine whether quality of care is lower for service members who experience a PCS or move from one MTF to another
- Assess whether quality of care differs between direct and purchased care
- Examine whether use of BHDP varies by service branch, region, MTFs, and providers.

Studies Requiring Additional Data Collection

- Understand service member and provider attitudes and use of BHDP to inform approaches to increase meaningful clinical use of outcome data
- Assess the impact of collecting outcome data only through the clinical context versus follow-up with patients via telephone or web
- Undertake qualitative and quantitative studies to better understand care processes and barriers to improving performance on quality measures
- Develop and test additional quality measures for PH care.

Summary

This report expands previous RAND research assessing the quality of care provided to active-component service members with PTSD or depression in the MHS. In this report, we analyzed three types of data (administrative, medical record, and symptom questionnaire) to assess performance using 30 quality measures (33 measures, when accounting for scores reported separately within a measure). We also used administrative data to describe patterns of care received by service members with PTSD or depression and examined variations in quality measure scores. Finally, we analyzed symptom questionnaire data to evaluate the relationship between quality of care and patient outcomes. MHS-wide performance across the quality measures was mixed. The MHS demonstrated excellent care in some areas; six measure scores (four for PTSD; two for depression) were at or above 90 percent (assessing PTSD symptom severity and PTSD and depression comorbidity and follow-up after MH hospitalization). In contrast, four PTSD measures and seven depression measures indicated that fewer than 50 percent of service members received the recommended care. In general, MHS-wide measure scores for PTSD were higher than those for depression. Analyzing variations in administrative data quality measure scores revealed several significant differences, with the largest variations by service branch, TRICARE region, pay grade, and age. These variations are important because they suggest that care is not consistently of high quality for all service members. No significant associations were found between receiving recommended care and improvements in patient symptom scores at six months, but the analyses were limited to a subgroup of patients with continued engagement and reassessment in behavioral health specialty care and a select group of quality measures. These findings highlight areas in which the MHS delivers excellent care, as well as areas that should be targeted for quality improvement. The results presented here should be useful to the MHS in identifying high-priority next steps to support continuous improvement in the care the MHS delivers to service members.

Bibliography

Agency for Healthcare Research and Quality, "Uses of Quality Measures," undated. As of September 12, 2015:
http://www.qualitymeasures.ahrq.gov/selecting-and-using/using.aspx

American Psychiatric Association, *Practice Guideline for the Treatment of Patients with Acute Stress Disorder and Posttraumatic Stress Disorder*, Washington, D.C.: American Pyschiatric Association, 2004.

———, *Diagnostic and Statistical Manual of Mental Disorders, Fifth Edition*, Arlington, Va.: American Psychiatric Association, 2013.

Association for Enterprise Information, "Behavioral Health Data Portal," undated. As of December 22, 2015:
http://www.afei.org/Awards/Documents/3_govt_BHDP_syn.pdf

Belsher, B. E., L. H. Jaycox, M. C. Freed, D. P. Evatt, X. Liu, L. A. Novak, D. Zatzick, R. M. Bray, and C. C. Engel, "Mental Health Utilization Patterns During a Stepped, Collaborative Care Effectiveness Trial for PTSD and Depression in the Military Health System," Medical Care, Vol. 54, No. 7, July 2016, pp. 706–713.

Benjamini, Yoav, and Yosef Hochberg, "Controlling the False Discovery Rate: A Practical and Powerful Approach to Multiple Testing," Journal of the Royal Statistical Society, Series B 57, Vol. 1, 1995, pp. 289–300.

Bisson, Jonathan, and Martin Andrew, "Psychological Treatment of Post-Traumatic Stress Disorder (PTSD)," The Cochrane Database of Systematic Reviews, No. 3, 2007, p. CD003388. As of December 22, 2015:
http://search.ebscohost.com/login.aspx?direct=true&db=cmedm&AN=17636720&site=ehost-live

Blais, Mark A., William R. Lenderking, Lee Baer, Ashley deLorell, Kathleen Peets, Linda Leahy, and Craig Burns, "Development and Initial Validation of a Brief Mental Health Outcome Measure," *Journal of Personality Assessment*, Vol. 73, No. 3, Dec, 1999, pp. 359–373.

Blakeley, Katherine, and Don J. Jansen, *Post-Traumatic Stress Disorder and Other Mental Health Problems in the Military: Oversight Issues for Congress*, Congressional Research Service, 7-5700, 2013. As of October 5, 2015:
https://www.fas.org/sgp/crs/natsec/R43175.pdf

Blanchard, Edward B., Jacqueline Jones-Alexander, Todd C. Buckley, and Catherine A. Forneris, "Psychometric Properties of the PTSD Checklist (PCL)," *Behaviour Research and Therapy*, Vol. 34, No. 8, 1996, pp. 669–673.

Bland, J. Martin, and Douglas G. Altman, "Statistics Notes: Some Examples of Regression Towards the Mean," *Bmj*, Vol. 309, No. 6957, 1994, p. 780.

Bliese, Paul D., Kathleen M. Wright, Amy B. Adler, Oscar Cabrera, Carl A. Castro, and Charles W. Hoge, "Validating the Primary Care Posttraumatic Stress Disorder Screen and the Posttraumatic Stress Disorder Checklist with Soldiers Returning from Combat," *Journal of Consulting and Clinical Psychology*, Vol. 76, No. 2, 2008, pp. 272–281. As of September 19, 2013: http://search.ebscohost.com/login.aspx?direct=true&db=cmedm&AN=18377123&site=ehost-live

Boyce, Maria B., and John P. Browne, "Does Providing Feedback on Patient-Reported Outcomes to Healthcare Professionals Result in Better Outcomes for Patients? A Systematic Review," *Quality of Life Research*, Vol. 22, No. 9, 2013, pp. 2265–2278.

Bradley, Katharine A., Emily C. Williams, Carol E. Achtmeyer, Bryan Volpp, Bonny J. Collins, and Daniel R. Kivlahan, "Implementation of Evidence-Based Alcohol Screening in the Veterans Health Administration," *American Journal of Managed Care*, Vol. 12, No. 10, 2006, pp. 597–606. As of September 19, 2013: https://www.researchgate.net/profile/Emily_Williams3/publication/6769494_Implementation_of_evidence-based_alcohol_screening_in_the_Veterans_Health_Administration/links/0912f50b7c1ed85800000000.pdf

Brown, Millard, Kelly Woolaway-Bickel, R. Laygo, and D. A. Nelson, "Clinical Outcomes in Army Behavioral Health Care Using the Behavioral Health Data Portal," Powerpoint presentation to American Psychological Association, 2015.

Burnett-Zeigler, Inger E., Paul Pfeiffer, Kara Zivin, Joseph E. Glass, Mark A. Ilgen, Heather A. Flynn, Karen Austin, and Stephen T. Chermack, "Psychotherapy Utilization for Acute Depression Within the Veterans Affairs Health Care System," *Psychological Services*, Vol. 9, No. 4, November 2012, pp. 325–335. As of September 19, 2013: http://www.ncbi.nlm.nih.gov/pubmed/22564035

Centers for Disease Control and Prevention, *Measuring Healthy Days*, Atlanta, Ga.: CDC, 2000. As of September 19, 2013: http://www.cdc.gov/hrqol/pdfs/mhd.pdf

Chen, Shih-Yin, Richard A. Hansen, Joel F. Farley, Bradley N. Gaynes, Joseph P. Morrissey, and Matthew L. Maciejewski, "Follow-up Visits by Provider Specialty for Patients with Major Depressive Disorder Initiating Antidepressant Treatment," *Psychiatric Services*, Vol. 61, No. 1, January 2010, pp. 81–85. As of September 19, 2013: http://www.ncbi.nlm.nih.gov/pubmed/20044424

Committee on the Assessment of Ongoing Efforts in the Treatment of Posttraumatic Stress Disorder, Board on the Health of Select Populations, Institute of Medicine, *Treatment for Posttraumatic Stress Disorder in Military and Veteran Populations: Final Assessment*, Washington, D.C.: National Academies Press, 2014. As of August 18, 2015: http://www.ncbi.nlm.nih.gov/books/NBK224879/

Cooper, Andrew A., Alexander C. Kline, Belinda P. M. Graham, Michele Bedard-Gilligan, Patricia G. Mello, Norah C. Feeny, and Lori A. Zoellner, "Homework 'Dose,' Type, and Helpfulness as Predictors of Clinical Outcomes in Prolonged Exposure for PTSD, Behavior Therapy," *Behavior Therapy*, 2016.

Cully, Jeffrey A., Laura Tolpin, Louise Henderson, Daniel Jimenez, Mark E. Kunik, and Laura A. Petersen, "Psychotherapy in the Veterans Health Administration: Missed Opportunities?" *Psychological Services*, Vol. 5, No. 4, 2008, pp. 320–331. As of August 18, 2015: http://www.ncbi.nlm.nih.gov/pmc/articles/PMC4145407/

Department of the Army Headquarters, "Behavioral Health Data Portal," Army Medical Command, undated. As of December 16, 2015: http://armymedicine.mil/Pages/BHDP.aspx

————, "OTSG/MEDCOM Policy Memo 11-061: MEDCOM Policy for Procedures Following Missed Behavioral Health (BH) Appointments," 2011.

————, "OTSG/MEDCOM Policy Memo 14-019: Inpatient and Emergency Department (ED) Aftercare," 2014a.

————, "OTSG/MEDCOM Policy Memo 14-094: Policy Guidance on the Assessment and Treatment of PTSD," 2014b.

Dixon, Lisa, Richard Goldberg, Virginia Iannone, Alicia Lucksted, Clayton Brown, Julie Kreyenbuhl, Lijuan Fang, and Wendy Potts, "Use of a Critical Time Intervention to Promote Continuity of Care After Psychiatric Inpatient Hospitalization," *Psychiatric Services*, Vol. 60, No. 4, 2009, pp. 451–458.

Dobscha, Steven K., Martha S. Gerrity, Kathryn Corson, Alison Bahr, and Nancy M. Cuilwik, "Measuring Adherence to Depression Treatment Guidelines in a VA Primary Care Clinic," *General Hospital Psychiatry*, Vol. 25, No. 4, 2003, pp. 230–237. As of August 7, 2003: http://www.sciencedirect.com/science/article/pii/S0163834303000203

DoD—*See* U.S. Department of Defense.

Engel, C. C., L. H. Jaycox, M. C. Freed, R. M. Bray, D. Brambilia, D. Zatzick, B. Litz, T. Tanielian, L. A. Novak, M. E. Lane, B. E. Belsher, K. L. Olmsted, D. P. Evatt, R. Vandermaas-Peeler, J. Unützer, and W. J. Katon, "Centrally Assisted Collaborative Telecare for Posttraumatic Stress Disorder and Depression Among Military Personnel Attending Primary Care: A Randomized Clinical Trial," JAMA Internal Medicine, Vol. 176, No. 7, July 2016, pp. 948–956.

Farmer, Carrie M., Katherine E. Watkins, Brad Smith, Susan M. Paddock, Abigail Woodroffe, Jacob Solomon, Melony E. Sorbero, Kimberly A. Hepner, Lanna Forrest, Lisa R. Shugarman, Cathy Call, and Harold A. Pincus, *Program Evaluation of VHA Mental Health Services: Medical Record Review Report*, Alexandria, Va.: Altarum Institute and RAND-University of Pittsburgh Health Institute, 2010.

Fischer, Ellen P., John F. McCarthy, Rosalinda V. Ignacio, Frederic C. Blow, Kristen L. Barry, Teresa J. Hudson, Richard R. Owen Jr., and Marcia Valenstein, "Longitudinal Patterns of Health System Retention Among Veterans with Schizophrenia or Bipolar Disorder," *Community Mental Health Journal*, Vol. 44, No. 5, October 1, 2008, pp. 321–330. As of August 8, 2015: http://dx.doi.org/10.1007/s10597-008-9133-z

Fournier, Jay C., Robert J. DeRubeis, Steven D. Hollon, Sona Dimidjian, Jay D. Amsterdam, Richard C. Shelton, and Jan Fawcett, "Antidepressant Drug Effects and Depression Severity: A Patient-Level Meta-Analysis," *JAMA: The Journal of the American Medical Association*, Vol. 303, No. 1, 2010, pp. 47–53. As of August 8, 2015: http://search.ebscohost.com/login.aspx?direct=true&db=cmedm&AN=20051569&site=ehost-live

Garin, Olatz, Jose L. Ayuso-Mateos, Josué Almansa, Marta Nieto, Somnath Chatterji, Gemma Vilagut, Jordi Alonso, Alarcos Cieza, Olga Svetskova, Helena Burger, Vittorio Racca, Carlo Francescutti, Eduard Vieta, Nenad Kostanjsek, Alberto Raggi, Matilde Leonardi, and Montse Ferrer, "Validation of the 'World Health Organization Disability Assessment Schedule, WHODAS-2' in Patients with Chronic Diseases," *Health and Quality of Life Outcomes*, Vol. 8, 2010, p. 51.

Garrison, Gregory M., Kurt B. Angstman, Stephen S. O'Connor, Mark D. Williams, and Timothy W. Lineberry, "Time to Remission for Depression with Collaborative Care Management (CCM) in Primary Care," *Journal of the American Board of Family Medicine*, Vol. 29, No. 1, January–February 2016, pp. 10–17. As of February 18, 2016: http://www.ncbi.nlm.nih.gov/pubmed/26769872

Glenberg, Alan J., Marlene P. Freeman, John C. Markowitz, Jerrold F. Rosenbaum, Michael E. Thase, Madhukar H. Trivedi, and Richard S. Van Rhoads, *Practice Guideline for the Treatment of Patients with Major Depressive Disorder*, Arlington, Va.: American Psychiatric Association, 2010.

Graham, J. W., "Missing Data Analysis: Making It Work in the Real World," *Annual Review of Psychology*, Vol. 60, 2009, pp. 549–576.

Greenberg, Greg A., Robert A. Rosenheck, and Alan Fontana, "Continuity of Care and Clinical Effectiveness: Treatment of Posttraumatic Stress Disorder in the Department of Veterans Affairs," *Journal of Behavioral Health Services and Research*, Vol. 30, No. 2, 2003, pp. 202–214.

Harding, Kelli Jane, A. John Rush, Melissa Arbuckle, Madhukar H. Trivedi, and Harold Alan Pincus, "Measurement-Based Care in Psychiatric Practice: A Policy Framework for Implementation," *Journal of Clinical Psychiatry*, Vol. 72, No. 8, 2011, pp. 1136–1143.

Harpaz-Rotem, Ilan, Daniel Libby, and Robert A. Rosenheck, "Psychotherapy Use in a Privately Insured Population of Patients Diagnosed with a Mental Disorder," *Social Psychiatry and Psychiatric Epidemiology*, Vol. 47, No. 11, 2012, pp. 1837–1844.

Haskell, Sally G., Kristin Mattocks, Joseph L. Goulet, Erin E. Krebs, Melissa Skanderson, Douglas Leslie, Amy C. Justice, Elizabeth M. Yano, and Cynthia Brandt, "The Burden of Illness in the First Year Home: Do Male and Female VA Users Differ in Health Conditions and Healthcare Utilization?" *Women's Health Issues*, Vol. 21, No. 1, January–February 2011, pp. 92–97. As of February 18, 2016:
http://www.ncbi.nlm.nih.gov/pubmed/21185994

Helmer, Drew A., Helena K. Chandler, Karen S. Quigley, Melissa Blatt, Ronald Teichman, and Gudrun Lange, "Chronic Widespread Pain, Mental Health, and Physical Role Function in OEF/OIF Veterans," *Pain Medicine*, Vol. 10, No. 7, October 2009, pp. 1174–1182. As of February 18, 2016:
http://www.ncbi.nlm.nih.gov/pubmed/19818029

Hepner, Kimberly A., Gregory L. Greenwood, Francisca Azocar, Jeanne Miranda, and M. Audrey Burnam, "Usual Care Psychotherapy for Depression in a Large Managed Behavioral Health Organization," *Administration and Policy in Mental Health and Mental Health Services Research*, Vol. 37, No. 3, 2009, pp. 270–278.

Hepner, Kimberly A., Carol P. Roth, Coreen Farris, Elizabeth M. Sloss, Grant Martsolf, Harold A. Pincus, Katherine E. Watkins, Caroline Epley, Daniel Mandel, Susan Hosek, and Carrie M. Farmer, *Measuring the Quality of Care for Psychological Health Conditions in the Military Health System: Candidate Measures for PTSD and Major Depression*, Santa Monica, Calif.: RAND Corporation, RR-464-OSD, 2015. As of February 18, 2016:
http://www.rand.org/pubs/research_reports/RR464.html

Hepner, Kimberly A., Melissa Rowe, Kathryn Rost, Scot C. Hickey, Cathy D. Sherbourne, Daniel E. Ford, Lisa S. Meredith, and Lisa V. Rubenstein, "The Effect of Adherence to Practice Guidelines on Depression Outcomes," *Annals of Internal Medicine*, Vol. 147, No. 5, 2007, pp. 320–329. As of February 18, 2016:
http://dx.doi.org/10.7326/0003-4819-147-5-200709040-00007

Hepner, Kimberly A., Elizabeth M. Sloss, Carol P. Roth, Heather Krull, Susan M. Paddock, Shaela Moen, Martha J. Timmer, and Harold A. Pincus, *Quality of Care for PTSD and Depression in the Military Health System: Phase 1 Report*, Santa Monica, Calif.: RAND Corporation, RR-978-OSD, 2016. As of February 18, 2016:
http://www.rand.org/pubs/research_reports/RR978.html

Hoge, Charles W., Jennifer L. Auchterlonie, and Charles S. Milliken, "Mental Health Problems, Use of Mental Health Services, and Attrition from Military Service After Returning from Deployment to Iraq or Afghanistan," *JAMA, The Journal of the American Medical Association*, Vol. 295, No. 9, March 1, 2006, pp. 1023–1032. As of February 18, 2016:
http://www.ncbi.nlm.nih.gov/pubmed/16507803

Hoge, Charles W., Sasha H. Grossman, Jennifer L. Auchterlonie, Lyndon A. Riviere, Charles S. Milliken, and Joshua E. Wilk, "PTSD Treatment for Soldiers After Combat Deployment: Low Utilization of Mental Health Care and Reasons for Dropout," *Psychiatric Services*, Vol. 65, No. 8, August 1, 2014, pp. 997–1004. As of Februry 18, 2016:
http://www.ncbi.nlm.nih.gov/pubmed/24788253

Hoge, Charles W., Christopher G. Ivany, Edward A. Brusher, Millard D. Brown, 3rd, John C. Shero, Amy B. Adler, Christopher H. Warner, and David T. Orman, "Transformation of Mental Health Care for U.S. Soldiers and Families During the Iraq and Afghanistan Wars: Where Science and Politics Intersect," *American Journal of Psychiatry*, November 10, 2015, pp. 334–343.

Horvitz-Lennon, Marcela, Katherine E. Watkins, Harold Alan Pincus, Lisa R. Shugarman, Brad Smith, Teryn Mattox, and Thomas E. Mannle, *Veterans Health Administration Mental Health Program Evaluation Technical Manual*, Santa Monica, Calif.: RAND Corporation, WR-682-VHA, 2009. As of October 1, 2013:
http://www.rand.org/pubs/working_papers/WR682

Hyland, Michael E., and Samantha C. Sodergren, "Development of a New Type of Global Quality of Life Scale, and Comparison of Performance and Preference for 12 Global Scales," *Quality of Life Research*, Vol. 5, No. 5, October 1996, pp. 469–480.

Institute of Medicine, *Crossing the Quality Chasm: A New Health System for the 21st Century*, Washington, D.C.: National Academies Press, 2001.

———, *Provision of Mental Health Counseling Services Under TRICARE*, Washington, D.C.: National Academies Press, 2010.

———, *Returning Home from Iraq and Afghanistan: Readjustment Needs of Veterans, Service Members, and Their Families*, Washington, D.C.: National Academies Press, 2013.

———, *Preventing Psychological Disorders in Service Members and Their Families: An Assessment of Programs*, Washington, D.C.: National Academies Press, 2014a.

———, *Treatment for Posttraumatic Stress Disorder in Military and Veteran Populations: Final Assessment*, Washington, D.C.: National Academies Press, 2014b.

———, *Psychosocial Interventions for Mental and Substance Use Disorders: A Framework for Establishing Evidence-Based Standards*, Washington, D.C.: National Academies Press., 2015.

Jain, Shaili, Mark A. Greenbaum, and Craig S. Rosen, "Do Veterans with Posttraumatic Stress Disorder Receive First-Line Pharmacotherapy? Results from the Longitudinal Veterans Health Survey," *Primary Care Companion to CNS Disorders*, Vol. 14, No. 2, 2012, p. PCC.11m01162. As of October 1, 2013:
http://www.ncbi.nlm.nih.gov/pmc/articles/PMC3425460/

Joint Commission, *Performance Measurement for Hospitals*, web portal, 2017. As of February 20, 2017:
http://www.jointcommission.org/accreditation/performance_measurementoryx.aspx

Jonas, Daniel E., Karen Cusack, Catherine A. Forneris, Tania M. Wilkins, Jeffrey Sonis, Jennifer Cook Middleton, Cynthia Feltner, Dane Meredith, Jamie Cavanaugh, Kimberly A. Brownley, Kristine Rae Olmsted, Amy Greenblatt, Amy Weil, and Bradley N. Gaynes, "Psychological and Pharmacological Treatments for Adults with Posttraumatic Stress Disorder (PTSD)," Comparative Effectiveness Review No. 92, AHRQ Publication No. 13-EHC011-EF, Rockville, Md.: Agency for Healthcare Research and Quality, April 2013. As of September 18, 2013: http://effectivehealthcare.ahrq.gov/ehc/products/347/1435/PTSD-adult-treatment-report-130403.pdf

Jordan, Neil, Min-Woong Sohn, Brian Bartle, Marcia Valenstein, Yuri Lee, and Todd A. Lee, "Association Between Chronic Illness Complexity and Receipt of Evidence-Based Depression Care," Medical Care, Vol. 52, 2014, pp. S126–S131.

Kilbourne, Amy M., Donna Keyser, and Harold A. Pincus, "Challenges and Opportunities in Measuring the Quality of Mental Health Care," Canadian Journal of Psychiatry, Vol. 55, No. 9, September 2010, pp. 549–557. As of September 18, 2013: http://www.ncbi.nlm.nih.gov/pubmed/20840802

Kim, Jae Kwang, and Jay J. Kim, "Nonresponse Weighting Adjustment Using Estimated Response Probability," Canadian Journal of Statistics, Vol. 35, No. 4, 2007, pp. 501–514.

Kroenke, Kurt, Robert L. Spitzer, and Janet B. W. Williams, "The PHQ-9: Validity of a Brief Depression Severity Measure," Journal of General Internal Medicine, Vol. 16, No. 9, 2001, pp. 606–613. As of September 18, 2013: http://dx.doi.org/10.1046/j.1525-1497.2001.016009606.x

Lagomasino, Isabel, Robert Daly, and Alan Stoudemire, "Medical Assessment of Patients Presenting with Psychiatric Symptoms in the Emergency Setting," Psychiatric Clinics of North America, Vol. 22, No. 4, 1999, pp. 819–850.

Löwe, Bernd, Jürgen Unützer, Christopher M. Callahan, Anthony J. Perkins, and Kurt Kroenke, "Monitoring Depression Treatment Outcomes with the Patient Health Questionnaire-9," Medical Care, Vol. 42, No. 12, 2004, pp. 1194–1201. As of September 18, 2013: http://search.ebscohost.com/login.aspx?direct=true&db=cmedm&AN=15550799&site=ehost-live

McGlynn, Elizabeth A., and John L. Adams, "What Makes a Good Quality Measure?" JAMA, The Journal of the American Medical Association, Vol. 312, No. 15, 2014, pp. 1517–1518. As of April 4, 2015: http://unmhospitalist.pbworks.com/w/file/fetch/88447109/jed140086.pdf

McHorney, Colleen A., John E. Ware Jr., and Anastasia E. Raczek, "The MOS 36-Item Short-Form Health Status Survey (SF-36), II: Psychometric and Clinical Tests of Validity in Measuring Physical and Mental Health Constructs," Medical Care, Vol. 31, No. 3, 1993.

Military Health System and Defense Health Agency, "Quality, Patient Safety and Access Information for MHS Patients," Falls Church, Va., 2016. As of July 20, 2016: http://www.health.mil/Military-Health-Topics/Access-Cost-Quality-and-Safety/Patient-Portal-for-MHS-Quality-Patient-Safety-and-Access-Information

Mitchell, Alex J., and Thomas Selmes, "Why Don't Patients Attend Their Appointments? Maintaining Engagement with Psychiatric Services," Advances in Psychiatric Treatment, Vol. 13, No. 6, November 1, 2007, pp. 423–434. As of April 4, 2015: http://apt.rcpsych.org/content/13/6/423.abstract

MN Community Measurement, "Previous Health Care Quality Reports," undated. As of April 4, 2015: http://mncm.org/previous-health-care-quality-reports/

————, "2013 Health Care Quality Report," 2013. As of March 15, 2015:
http://mncm.org/wp-content/uploads/2014/02/2013-HCQR-Final-2.4.2014.pdf

————, "2014 Health Care Quality Report," 2014. As of March 15, 2015:
http://mncm.org/wp-content/uploads/2015/01/2014-Health-Care-Quality-Report-FINAL-1.27.2015.
pdf

————, "2015 Health Care Quality Report," 2015. As of April 4, 2016:
http://mncm.org/wp-content/uploads/2015/11/2015-Health-Care-Quality-Report-Final1.pdf

Moncrieff, J., S. Wessely, and R. Hardy, "Active Placebos versus Antidepressants for Depression,"
Cochrane Database of Systematic Reviews, No. 1, 2004, p. CD003012. As of April 4, 2016:
http://search.ebscohost.com/login.aspx?direct=true&db=cmedm&AN=14974002&site=ehost-live

Monson, Candice M., Jaimie L. Gradus, Yinong Young-Xu, Paula P. Schnurr, Jennifer L. Price, and
Jeremiah A. Schumm, "Change in Posttraumatic Stress Disorder Symptoms: Do Clinicians and
Patients Agree?," *Psychological Assessment*, Vol. 20, No. 2, 2008, pp. 131–138. As of April 4, 2016:
http://search.ebscohost.com/login.aspx?direct=true&db=cmedm&AN=18557690&site=ehost-live

Moriarty, David, Mathew Zack, and Rosemarie Kobau, "The Centers for Disease Control and
Prevention's Healthy Days Measures—Population Tracking of Perceived Physical and Mental Health
over Time," *Health and Quality of Life Outcomes*, Vol. 1, No. 1, 2003, p. 37.

Mott, Juliette M., Natalie E. Hundt, Shubhada Sansgiry, Joseph Mignogna, and Jeffrey A. Cully,
"Changes in Psychotherapy Utilization Among Veterans with Depression, Anxiety, and PTSD,"
Psychiatric Services, Vol. 65, No. 1, 2014, pp. 106–112. As of April 4, 2016:
http://ps.psychiatryonline.org/doi/abs/10.1176/appi.ps.201300056

National Center for PTSD, "Using the PTSD Checklist," fact sheet, Washington, D.C., U.S.
Department of Veterans Affairs, 2012. As of May 15, 2013:
http://www.ptsd.va.gov/professional/pages/assessments/ptsd-checklist.asp

National Committee for Quality Assurance, "State of Health Care Quality 2008," 2008. As of April
4, 2016:
https://www.ncqa.org/Portals/0/Newsroom/SOHC/SOHC_08.pdf

————, "2015 State of Health Care Quality: Antidepressant Medication Management," 2015a. As of
April 5, 2016:
http://www.ncqa.org/report-cards/health-plans/state-of-health-care-quality/2015-table-of-contents/
antidepressant

————, "2015 State of Health Care Quality: Follow-up After Hospitalization for Mental Illness,"
2015b. As of April 4, 2016:
http://www.ncqa.org/report-cards/health-plans/state-of-health-care-quality/2015-table-of-contents

National Quality Forum, "Quality Positioning System," database, 2013a. As of January 2, 2015:
http://www.qualityforum.org/QPS/QPSTool.aspx

————, "NQF #0104 Adult Major Depressive Disorder (MDD): Suicide Risk Assessment," 2014a.
As of April 4, 2016:
http://www.qualityforum.org/QPS

————, "NQF #0105 Anti-Depressant Medication Management (AMM)," 2014b. As of March 14,
2016:
http://www.qualityforum.org/QPS

————, "NQF #0711 Depression Remission at Six Months," 2015a. As of March 3, 2016:
http://www.qualityforum.org/QPS

————, "NQF #0712 Depression Utilization of the PHQ-9 Tool," 2015b. As of March 15, 2016:
http://www.qualityforum.org/QPS

————, "Patient Safety," web page, 2017a. As of February 15, 2017:
http://www.qualityforum.org/Topics/Patient_Safety.aspx

————, "Disparities," web page, 2017b. As of February 15, 2017:
http://www.qualityforum.org/Topics/Disparities.aspx

Oxman, Thomas E., Allen J. Dietrich, John W. Williams, Charles C. Engel, Matthew Friedman, Paula Schnurr, Stanley Rosenberg, and Sheila L. Barry, *RESPECT-Mil Primary Care Clinician's Manual: 3CM-LLC*, 2008.

Parast, L., B. Doyle, C. L. Damberg, K. Shetty, D. A. Ganz, N. S. Wenger, and P. G. Shekelle, "Challenges in Assessing the Process-Outcome Link in Practice," *Journal of General Internal Medicine*, Vol. 30, No. 3, March 2015, pp. 359–364. As of March 15, 2016:
http://www.ncbi.nlm.nih.gov/pubmed/25564435

Pfeiffer, Paul N., Dara Ganoczy, Nicholas W. Bowersox, John F. McCarthy, Frederic C. Blow, and Marcia Valenstein, "Depression Care Following Psychiatric Hospitalization in the Veterans Health Administration," *American Journal of Managed Care*, Vol. 17, No. 9, September 2011, pp. e358–e364. As of March 15, 2016:
http://www.ncbi.nlm.nih.gov/pubmed/21902443

Pincus, Harold A., Brigitta Spaeth-Rublee, and Katherine E. Watkins, "Analysis and Commentary: The Case for Measuring Quality in Mental Health and Substance Abuse Care," *Health Affairs* (Millwood), Vol. 30, No. 4, April 2011, pp. 730–736. As of March 15, 2016:
http://www.ncbi.nlm.nih.gov/pubmed/21471495

Posner, Kelly, Gregory K. Brown, Barbara Stanley, David A. Brent, Kseniya V. Yershova, Maria A. Oquendo, Glenn W. Currier, Glenn A. Melvin, Laurence Greenhill, Sa Shen, and J. John Mann, "The Columbia–Suicide Severity Rating Scale: Initial Validity and Internal Consistency Findings from Three Multisite Studies with Adolescents and Adults," *American Journal of Psychiatry*, Vol. 168, No. 12, December 2011, pp. 1266–1277.

Rabin, Rosalind, and Frank de Charro, "EQ-5D: A Measure of Health Status from the EuroQol Group," *Annals of Medicine*, Vol. 33, No. 5, 2001, pp. 337–343.

Ramchand, Rajeev, Rena Rudavsky, Sean Grant, Terri L. Tanielian, and Lisa Jaycox, "Prevalence of, Risk Factors for, and Consequences of Posttraumatic Stress Disorder and Other Mental Health Problems in Military Populations Deployed to Iraq and Afghanistan," *Current Psychiatry Reports*, Vol. 17, No. 5, May 2015, p. 37. As of March 15, 2016:
http://www.ncbi.nlm.nih.gov/pubmed/25876141

Saunders, John B., Olaf G. Aasland, Thomas F. Babor, Juan R. De la Fuente, and Marcus Grant, "Development of the Alcohol Use Disorders Identification Test (AUDIT): WHO Collaborative Project on Early Detection of Persons with Harmful Alcohol Consumption-II," *Addiction*, Vol. 88, No. 6, 1993, pp. 791–804.

Sheehan, David V., Kathy Harnett-Sheehan, and Balaibail Ashok Raj, "The Measurement of Disability," *International Clinical Psychopharmacology*, Vol. 11, 1996, pp. 89–95.

Shin, Hana J., Mark A. Greenbaum, Shaili Jain, and Craig S. Rosen, "Associations of Psychotherapy Dose and SSRI or SNRI Refills with Mental Health Outcomes Among Veterans with PTSD," *Psychiatric Services*, Vol. 65, No. 10, October 2014, pp. 1244–1248. As of March 15, 2016:
http://www.ncbi.nlm.nih.gov/pubmed/24981643

Sklar, Marisa, Andrew Sarkin, Todd Gilmer, and Erik Groessl, "The Psychometric Properties of the Illness Management and Recovery Scale in a Large American Public Mental Health System," *Psychiatry Research*, Vol. 199, No. 3, October 30, 2012, pp. 220–227.

Smith, Bruce W., Jeanne Dalen, Kathryn Wiggins, Erin Tooley, Paulette Christopher, and Jennifer Bernard, "The Brief Resilience Scale: Assessing the Ability to Bounce Back," *International Journal of Behavioral Medicine*, Vol. 15, No. 3, 2008, pp. 194–200.

Sorbero, Melony E., Thomas E. Mannle, Brad Smith, Katherine E. Watkins, Abigail Woodroffe, Susan M. Paddock, Lisa R. Shugarman, E. Dela Cruz, Jacob Solomon, Q. Burkhart, Teryn Mattox, and Harold A. Pincus, *Program Evaluation of VHA Mental Health Services: Administrative Data Report*, Alexandria, Va.: Altarum Institute and RAND–University of Pittsburgh Health Institute, 2010.

Spoont, Michele, Maureen Murdoch, James Hodges, and Sean Nugent, "Treatment Receipt by Veterans After a PTSD Diagnosis in PTSD, Mental Health, or General Medical Clinics," *Psychiatric Services*, Vol. 61, No. 1, 2010, pp. 58–63.

Steenkamp, Maria M., Brett T. Litz, Charles W. Hoge, and Charles R. Marmar, "Psychotherapy for Military-Related PTSD: A Review of Randomized Clinical Trials," *JAMA, The Journal of the American Medical Association*, Vol. 314, No. 5, August 4, 2015, pp. 489–500. As of December 16, 2015:
http://www.ncbi.nlm.nih.gov/pubmed/26241600

Tanielian, Terri L., and Lisa Jaycox, *Invisible Wounds of War: Psychological and Cognitive Injuries, Their Consequences, and Services to Assist Recovery*, Santa Monica, Calif.: RAND Corporation, MG-720-CCF, 2008. As of December 16, 2015:
http://www.rand.org/pubs/monographs/MG720.html

Trangle, Michael, Benita Dieperink, Thomas Gabert, Bob Haight, Britta Lindvall, Jay Mitchell, Heidi Novak, D. Rich, David Rossmiller, Linda Setterlund, and Kristin Somers, *Major Depression in Adults in Primary Care*, Bloomington, Minn.: Institute for Clinical Systems, 2012.

U.S. Army Task Force on Behavioral Health, "Corrective Action Plan," January 2013. As of May 13, 2015:
http://www.asamra.army.mil/docs/ATFBH%20Corrective%20Action%20Plan%205%20March%2013.pdf

U.S. Department of Defense, "HA Policy 02-016: Military Health System Definitions of Quality in Health Care," Military Health System official website, Defense Health Agency, Falls Church, Va., May 9, 2002. As of February 18, 2016:
http://www.health.mil/Policies?&query=02-016

———, *Military Treatment Facility Mental Health Clinical Outcomes Guidance Memorandum*, Washington, D.C., Assistant Secretary of Defense, Affairs, Manpower and Reserve, 2013. As of August 18, 2015:
http://www.dcoe.mil/Libraries/Documents/MentalHealthClinicalOutcomesGuidance_Woodson.pdf

———, "Build Resilience to Maximize Mission Readiness," Real Warriors website, Defense Centers of Excellence, 2014a. As of August 18, 2015:
http://realwarriors.net/active/treatment/resilience.php

———, "Evaluation of the TRICARE Program, Fiscal Year 2014 Report to Congress," 2014b. As of August 18, 2015:
http://health.mil/Military-Health-Topics/Access-Cost-Quality-and-Safety/
Health-Care-Program-Evaluation/Annual-Evaluation-of-the-TRICARE-Program?type=Reports

————, "Military Health System Review: Final Report to the Secretary of Defense," Military Health System official website, Defense Health Agency, Falls Church, Va., 2014c. As of August 18, 2015:
http://www.health.mil/Military-Health-Topics/Access-Cost-Quality-and-Safety/MHS-Review

————, "Evaluation of the TRICARE Program: Access, Cost and Quality, Fiscal Year 2015 Report to Congress," 2015. As of August 18, 2015:
http://health.mil/Military-Health-Topics/Access-Cost-Quality-and-Safety/
Health-Care-Program-Evaluation/Annual-Evaluation-of-the-TRICARE-Program?type=Reports

————, Report to Armed Services Committees of the Senate and House of Representatives, *Section 729 of the National Defense Authorization Act for Fiscal Year 2016 (Public Law 114-92), Plan for Development of Procedures to Measure Data on Mental Health Care Provided by the Department of Defense*, September 2016.

U.S. Department of Defense Deployment Health Clinical Center, and Post-Deployment Health Guidance Expert Panel, *Recommendations for Monitoring Metrics: DoD/VA Practice Guideline for Post-Deployment Health Evaluation and Management*, 2001. As of September 13, 2013:
http://www.pdhealth.mil/guidelines/downloads/view/3/2_recommendations_for_metrics.pdf

U.S. Department of Defense National Center for Telehealth and Technology, "DoDSER—Department of Defense Suicide Event Report: Calendar Year 2014 Annual Report," Defense Centers of Excellence for Psychological Health and Traumatic Brain Injury, 2016. As of February 18, 2016:
http://t2health.dcoe.mil/sites/default/files/CY-2014-DoDSER-Annual-Report.pdf

U.S. Department of Defense Office of the Deputy Assistant Secretary of Defense (Military Community and Family Policy), "2013 Demographics: Profile of the Military Community," 2014d. As of August 12, 2015:
http://download.militaryonesource.mil/12038/MOS/Reports/2013-Demographics-Report.pdf

U.S. Department of Defense Working Group on Common Mental Health Metrics, *Recommendations for Common Metrics for Assessing Progress in Addressing Psychological Health Problems*, Rockville, Md.: Substance Abuse and Mental Health Services Administration, U.S. Department of Health and Human Services, 2014e.

U.S. Department of Defense Deployment Health Clinical Center, and Post-Deployment Health Guidance Expert Panel, "Recommendations for Monitoring Metrics: DoD/VA Practice Guideline for Post-Deployment Health Evaluation and Management," 2001. As of April 4, 2015:
http://www.pdhealth.mil/guidelines/downloads/view/3/2_recommendations_for_metrics.pdf

U.S. Department of Defense and U.S. Department of Veterans Affairs, "DoD and VA Take New Steps to Support the Mental Health Needs of Service Members and Veterans," press release No. NR-446-14, August 26, 2014. As of March 15, 2015:
http://www.defense.gov/News/News-Releases/News-Release-View/Article/605153/
dod-and-va-take-new-steps-to-support-the-mental-health-needs-of-service-members

U.S. Department of Veterans Affairs, "VA/DoD Clinical Practice Guidelines: Safety Plan Worksheet," 2014. As of March 15, 2015:
http://www.healthquality.va.gov/guidelines/MH/srb/PatientSafetyPlanWorksheet110614v1.pdf

U.S. Department of Veterans Affairs and U.S. Department of Defense, "VA/DoD Clinical Practice Guideline: for Management of Major Depressive Disorder," Version 2.0–2008, Management of MDD Working Group, May, 2009. As of September 10, 2013:
http://www.healthquality.va.gov/mdd/MDD_FULL_3c1.pdf

———, "VA/DoD Clinical Practice Guideline for Management of Post-Traumatic Stress Disorder," Version 2.0–2010, Management of Post-Traumatic Stress Working Group, October 2010. As of September 10, 2013:
http://www.healthquality.va.gov/PTSD-full-2010c.pdf

———, "VA/DoD Clinical Practice Guideline for Assessment and Management of Patients at Risk for Suicide," Version 1.0, Assessment and Management of Risk for Suicide Working Group, June 2013. As of September 24, 2013:
http://www.healthquality.va.gov/guidelines/MH/srb/VADODCP_SuicideRisk_Full.pdf

———, "VA/DoD Clinical Practice Guideline for Management of Major Depressive Disorder," Version 3.0–2016, Mangement of Major Depressive Disorder Working Group, April 2016. As of May 27, 2016:
http://www.healthquality.va.gov/guidelines/mh/mdd/index.asp

U.S. Government Accountability Office, *VA Health Care: Improvements Needed in Monitoring Antidepressant Use in Major Depressive Disorder and in Increasing Accuracy of Suicide Data*, report to the chairman, Subcommittee on Oversight and Investigations, Committee on Veterans Affairs, U.S. House of Representatives, GAO-15-55, Washington, D.C., 2014. As of May 27, 2016:
http://www.gao.gov/assets/670/666842.pdf

U.S. Secretary of Defense, "Military Health System Action Plan for Access, Quality of Care, and Patient Safety," memorandum, 2014. As of March 15, 2016:
http://www.defense.gov/home/features/2014/0614_healthreview/docs/SD_Action_Memo.pdf

VA—*See* U.S. Department of Veterans Affairs.

Watkins, Katherine E., Harold A. Pincus, Susan Paddock, Brad Smith, Abigail Woodroffe, Carrie M. Farmer, Melony E. Sorbero, Marcela Horvitz-Lennon, Thomas Mannle, and Kimberly A. Hepner, "Care for Veterans with Mental and Substance Use Disorders: Good Performance, But Room to Improve on Many Measures," *Health Affairs*, Vol. 30, No. 11, 2011, pp. 2194–2203.

Weathers, Frank W., Brett T. Litz, Terence M. Keane, Patrick A. Palmieri, Brian P. Marx, and Paula P. Schnurr, "The PTSD Checklist for DSM-5 (PCL-5)," National Center for PTSD, U.S. Department of Veterans Affairs, 2013. As of March 29, 2015:
http://www.ptsd.va.gov/professional/assessment/adult-sr/ptsd-checklist.asp

Williams, Edwin R., and Suzanne Moore Shepherd, "Medical Clearance of Psychiatric Patients," *Emergency Medicine Clinics of North America*, Vol. 18, No. 2, 2000, pp. 185–198.

Woodson, Jonathan, Assistant Secretary of Defense for Health Affairs, "Military Treatment Facility Mental Health Clinical Outcomes Guidance," memorandum, 2013. As of March 29, 2015:
http://www.pdhealth.mil/ehc/OASDmemo_dtd09sep13.pdf

———, "MHS Leadership Message—Transparency, Military Health System monthly message, January 9, 2015a. As of March 10, 2015:
http://www.airforcemedicine.af.mil/News/Article/582461/mhs-leadership-message-transparency

———, *Prepared Statement of Jonathan Woodson, M.D., Assistant Secretary of Defense (Health Affairs) and Surgeons General of the Military Departments Before the House Armed Services Committee Subcommittee on Military Personnel*, June 11, 2015b. As of March 15, 2016:
http://www.med.navy.mil/bumed/comms/Documents/Congressional%20Testimonies/2015%20Hearings/06-11-2015%20HASC%20-%20MCRMC%20Recs%20-%20Woodson%20%20SGs%20FINAL.pdf

———, "The Military Health System as a High Reliability Organization," memo to military health system leadership, 2016.

Yehuda, Rachel, and Charles W. Hoge, "The Meaning of Evidence-Based Treatments for Veterans with Posttraumatic Stress Disorder," *JAMA Psychiatry*, February 17, 2016. As of March 15, 2016: http://www.ncbi.nlm.nih.gov/pubmed/26886229